THE MAGIC ABOUT PAIN

HOW FACING YOUR PAIN CAN TRANSFORM YOUR LIFE

Annabelle Breuer-Udo

authorHOUSE®

AuthorHouse™
1663 Liberty Drive
Bloomington, IN 47403
www.authorhouse.com
Phone: 1 (800) 839-8640

Published by AuthorHouse 11/12/2018

ISBN: 978-1-5462-6623-5 (sc)
ISBN: 978-1-5462-6621-1 (hc)
ISBN: 978-1-5462-6622-8 (e)

Library of Congress Control Number: 2018913180

Print information available on the last page.

*Any people depicted in stock imagery provided by Getty Images are models,
and such images are being used for illustrative purposes only.
Certain stock imagery © Getty Images.*

This book is printed on acid-free paper.

*Because of the dynamic nature of the Internet, any web addresses or links contained in
this book may have changed since publication and may no longer be valid. The views
expressed in this work are solely those of the author and do not necessarily reflect the
views of the publisher, and the publisher hereby disclaims any responsibility for them.*

Contents

For my husband, Okokon, who always believes in me and supports me on my unique soul path and journey! Thank you for walking the path with me in this life and being committed to a life created from the truest essence and self.

CHAPTER

1

ANOTHER DAY WITH NECK AND BACK PAIN

ON MONDAY MORNING, Anna wakes up with severe neck and back pain again. Her night was awful. She is restless and feels like a truck ran over her. She wonders, *How will I survive this day and this week?* And she talks to herself. "I have to get up and get Lisa and Jason ready for school. I hope they will hurry up, and we will not have these endless discussions about what to wear like almost every day. We need to leave right on time. I have a meeting with my boss. I wish Steve were here to help me, but he had to leave early this morning for a business trip." Pressure and stress are sitting in Anna's neck and back. She carries a lot on her shoulders, and this pain is penetrating her so much that her quality of life is very much affected.

Anna puts all her energy into her children, her team at work, her coaching business, and her marriage. Her life at work seems to be okay from the outside, and her relationship with her husband does too. She has seen doctors and specialists, and they have told her she is healthy. She went to see a chiropractor and some massage therapists, but they are not helping her for the long term. After any treatment, the pain may go away or lessen for a few days, but it comes back. This pain is penetrating and frustrating her. She feels exhaustion in her whole body, and her energy level is low most of the time. She is not as focused at work or on the things she needs to do. And her nights are horrible. She is not sleeping well; she is turning from side to side and feeling restless. In the morning, it is hard to get up and get out of bed.

What if this pain never goes away? she thinks. *I feel desperate, and I don't know what to do anymore. My biggest dream is getting rid of this pain and feeling much better.*

I hear Anna, and I understand where she is—and where you are—in life.

The cost of staying in this pain and not solving this problem may be severe. If nothing changes, your health could be affected later on. Worst case, you may want to numb the pain through different things, such as taking one or two more glasses of wine every evening. You may end up eating more and more to distract yourself from the pain. You may take painkillers or increase the doses of painkillers that affect your liver, kidney, and intestines. You may exaggerate your sports or running habits to have a few minutes without pain, although the pain is much worse after running. The patterns of distraction or addiction might continue. The more you are trapped in this circle of repeating destructive patterns, the harder it is to find a way out.

As hard as you have tried, you are still in the same place. You are trying to find a way out. You know it is not right to numb your pain or ignore it, but it makes you feel frustrated, desperate, and hopeless. It is not fun at all.

You may have tried so many things to get better and not know what else to do since nothing seems to work over the long term. There are days when the tension in your back is high and the pressure in your neck is unbearable. Therefore, you react less patiently with your children, and your relationship with your husband may be affected too.

On painful days, your mood is affected. At work, your team members notice you are very impatient. In your coaching sessions with your clients, you are not 100 percent present. On top of this, your boss is telling you that you should be happier at work and less emotional. Emotions have to stay at home. The pain limits you in the way of you are being. Playing with your kids, traveling, and even sitting at your desk are hard.

There is no way out, Anna thinks.

I get you where you are, and I can feel your pain!

If you identify with Anna, you know how hard it is to break this cycle. You feel trapped because you're not living the life you were supposed to live, although everything seems to be okay from the outside. You are aware that it sometimes affects your mood and your relationships with your husband, your children, your boss, your team members, and your clients. There are days when you are in fear of losing your job or your husband. I know these days and these feelings. You are not alone!

There is a difference between acute pain and chronic pain. Acute pain lasts temporarily, and chronic pain is persistent. Chronic pain stays for days, weeks, months, or even years. If you suffer from chronic pain, whether it is chronic neck or back pain or emotional pain, you are not alone!

Chronic Pain Statistics

- The Institute of Medicine of the National Academies reports that one hundred million Americans suffer from chronic pain.
- More than 1.5 billion people worldwide suffer from chronic pain, including eight to sixteen million Germans.
- Three out of four Americans have personally suffered from chronic pain or have a close friend or family member who has experienced it.
- Chronic pain affects more Americans than diabetes, cancer, and heart issues combined.
- Lower back pain is the most common type of chronic pain; more than twenty-six million Americans between the ages of twenty and sixty-four are affected.
- About forty-two million American adults have pain or physical distress that interrupts their sleep a few nights a week.
- Four out of ten people with chronic pain report the impact on their enjoyment of life, including impeding their mood, sleep, or ability to work.
- In Germany, 39 percent of people with chronic pain report the negative impact on their family members and friends, 50 percent say it has an impact on their employment status, 21 percent report they feel isolated due to their chronic pain, and 77 percent feel depressed due to chronic pain.

The four most common types of chronic pain in America are:

- lower back pain (27 percent)
- migraine pain or massive headaches (15 percent)
- neck pain (15 percent)
- facial pain (4 percent)

Apparently, women experience the common types of chronic pain more than men.

After those real and sobering numbers, I want to take you on another trip. I want you to dream about letting go of this pain and feeling much better. I want a solution that you can fit into your busy life, and I want to help you heal the pain for good.

Just pause here and think for a moment. What would a world without neck and back pain look like? Imagine your new world with the problem solved. You wake up several mornings without pain, fully rested and recovered, and start a new day with anticipation. You can travel without any problems, playing with your children is fun, and sitting at a desk is not a problem at all. Your focus on things at work, your daily life is sharp, and you are 100 percent present with your coaching clients and team members. Your boss gives you positive feedback on your powerful impact. Does it sound like something you have dreamed about?

Many of my clients were desperately in pain for a while, but they were not willing to commit to walking a different path. And that is fine. There are people who are standing on one side of the bridge where it looks dark and feels cold and painful, and they are suffering. They are not ready for this journey. Since their souls are not ready for this journey, they keep standing on that side.

Other people have started crossing the bridge. They are walking out of the dark, cold place of suffering and pain and moving toward the side of warmth, light, relief, and no pain. I meet them on the first third, halfway, or the last third. They are looking for help and support because they have decided to make a difference in their lives, but they need somebody who can give guidance to them on their hero journey.

In this book, you will get guidance on your hero journey. This book will open the door and show you change in a few steps. You will find the reasons that are causing your pain. You will find exercises and tools to master and nourish yourself and much more.

I encourage you and empower you to open your heart to this process, and I hope I will meet you somewhere on the bridge to guide you on your hero journey!

I want to talk to you about fear. You may have fears about losing your job, your clients, or your husband. You may have concerns and fears about what will happen if you walk this talk and commit to making a difference in your life. You might be afraid of letting go of control and not knowing what will happen to you after this process. You might not trust the process yet.

What is the most significant fear that is holding you back from facing your pain differently?

CHAPTER
2

━━━━━━━━━━━━━━━━━━━━●

MY STORY AND WHY
I WROTE THIS BOOK

There is no coming to consciousness without pain.
—Carl Gustav Jung

PAIN HAS BEEN an important ally, force, and wise guide in my life. It shows me so much, and I can see the benefits from another perspective when it shows up again. It does not show up very often anymore. It shows up in times of change, when I'm stuck, when I'm struggling with something, or in times of transition and unknowns. It knocks on my door softly, and if I do not listen to it, it becomes loud. I see the pain more as an ally than as an enemy. The pain is a navigator in life for me. The pain has moved me to find myself again and connect with my core, my truest Self, and my soul. It has helped me figure out who I am and to see what I want and need. It supported me in learning to set healthy boundaries and say no.

The pain and stress in your body is trying to wake you up and pay attention—maybe for the first time in your life. It is time to break the cycle of pain and stress and take time for yourselves. It is time to feel your body and listen to the screams of your soul. It is time to stop giving and giving and giving. It is time to stop putting all the energy in outside projects, family, and work. Instead of giving to others first, it is time to give the oxygen mask to yourself first—except for children. It is time to fill up the glass and give from an overflowing glass instead of giving from an empty glass. It is time to make a difference and experience how it feels to receive and stay in receiving and celebrating life. It is time to drive on a balanced wheel of life instead of an edgy one.

All of this can be found in my book, and I'm happy to help you feel better and stop living in pain and stress. I'm happy to walk the path beside you and guide the way. I would love for you to cross the bridge from the darker, painful, stressful cold place and move to the side of light, warmth, joy, love, relief, and softness.

Just because you have not found a way to get out of your pain and stress yet doesn't mean that it is impossible. Don't give up!

Anna's story is the story of so many of us. So many people suffer from neck pain, back pain, and other chronic pain. They wake up in pain and go to bed with pain. I lived in pain for many years in my twenties and thirties. It started just after I founded my osteopathy and physiotherapy practice with a colleague. It was an exciting time. I was a self-employed entrepreneur and was responsible for a small practice team. When started to study osteopathy, naturopathy, and psychotherapy, I married my first husband. All of it was running at the same time, and it was very challenging. I put all my energy into my business, studying, and my marriage. I had a high standard and thought I needed to manage and organize everything on my own.

From my point of view, everything was great. My life was great, but lower back pain was constantly in the background. I ignored it most of the time because I thought I needed to function at work and in my marriage. I believed there was no time to be sick. I had a business, I had to finish my study of osteopathy, and I had to be 100 percent present in my marriage all the time.

A friend asked if I had ever been to a doctor or specialist for the pain, and I said no. I was afraid that a doctor would say, "You have XYZ, and you need to stop your career and close your business here and now."

I took the question seriously and consulted doctors and specialists. All of them gave me the green light. I was healthy. There was nothing wrong medically. I was happy to hear the results, but I was confused because I wanted to know where the pain was coming from. My intuition told me there had to be a reason for pain.

As an expert in the medical world, it was especially important for me to find the reason. I had started my career in alternative holistic medicine, combining Western and Eastern medicine, and holistic health and well-being. My clients were in pain every day. It triggered my curiosity, and I felt an urge to figure out where the pain was coming from.

I looked for reasons and found explanations and ways to alleviate it. I tried out different massage treatments and physiotherapists, but nothing worked. It only reduced the pain for a few days, and then it came back. It was alleviating the symptoms without solving the root of the problem. There were days I could deal very well with it, but on other days, I felt covered in pain. I was not fully present at work or with my clients or colleagues. I could not really focus on studying or my marriage. I was running low on energy. I did my best as much as possible, but I was absorbed in the pain.

I consulted an osteopath, and I felt an improvement. For the first time, my pain stayed away for more than a week. I was hopeful and motivated. After a long time looking for a way out, I finally felt some changes in my body. In addition to frequently consulting the osteopath, I also started practicing yoga.

At the beginning of my first yoga session, the instructor announced that we would do some postures, breathing, and meditation techniques that were related to our heart chakras. At this time, I had no clue what chakra work was. I had little experience with meditation and breathing techniques. I was curious and followed the instructions. While I was focusing and breathing in one posture, I suddenly broke out in tears. It was an overwhelming feeling, and I had no control over it. I did not understand why I was crying when everything in my life was okay from the outside.

Looking back, I understand what was happening. The yoga session went very deep, and the results were huge. For days, my body felt different. The pain was far away and went naturally into the background. I felt like something opened on an emotional level.

I was a bit scared and I thought I did not need to give the experience too much attention. I had found a way to release the pain, and I only needed to continue with the osteopath every so often and practice yoga every week. Osteopathy and yoga have had a very positive impact on my pain and quality of life.

I took time out of my busy life to take care of healing the pain. I was in wonder of this special yoga session and the emotional experience that had a tremendous impact on my pain. I came to a point where I was brave enough to find out more. Yoga had a bigger influence on me than osteopathy. The yoga affected my physical body and my emotional body. Some of my hidden and suppressed emotions were surfacing. They needed attention, which was related to my physical pain. Staying in this emotional zone of discomfort was very uncomfortable.

In my five years of studying osteopathy, naturopathy, and psychotherapy, some of my teachers recommended inner emotional work, Shadow work, healing, and cleaning up your inner house. You can only go so far and deep with your clients as far as you have gone on your path of transformation. We all have hidden traumatic experiences. Everyone has experienced at least one traumatic experience. It does not matter if it was a small trauma or a big trauma. These experiences keep running in our cell memories and tissues if we do not face them and heal them. The Shock/Developmental Trauma I have experienced in my early life was partly running in my cell memories and causing pain and stress in my body. My first yoga instructor said, "Your issue lies in your tissue." And it is said that our very first trauma in life is our birth trauma.

I took the advice from my osteopathy teacher seriously and began doing inner work and healing. A life and business coach who was very experienced working with emotions, healing the inner child, and shadow work accompanied me on that path. It was the first time I experienced coaching.

At the beginning of my coaching journey, I was scared because I did not know what would happen and what would come out. I was curious, and I was guided by something that told me I had to do it to feel better, to get rid of the pain, and to move on in life. After starting with coaching and weekly yoga, the lower back pain and neck pain were no longer an issue. Other issues that were strongly related to my body pain surfaced: my relationship with my first husband and my work, my relationship with my colleagues, the systems at work, and my hidden dreams. A lot of things were suppressed, repressed, and held back, which caused stress, pressure, and pain.

I learned to understand that the pain in my body was the language of my soul talking to me and asking, "Are you still on the right path in your life? Are you living the life you want to live—or are you living somebody else's life? Are you still following your heart or are you betraying yourself and living a life that it is not yours?"

The combination of coaching and yoga was excellent for me! It encouraged me to transform and heal the pain. The pain was not at the forefront anymore, but sometimes it was hard to face all the issues contained in the pain. It opened some emotional pain, and I was taught that real change is an emotional process. I fully agree with this view, and in my experience, real change is an emotional process.

I encourage everyone to walk the path. It is worth it. Would I do it again? Yes, yes, and yes! In the same order? I think I would start with coaching much earlier. I waited too long because I was afraid to face the issues. I was not educated in talking about emotions and showing vulnerability. I thought, *I can do it on my own. I can figure it out all on my own. I do not need help. The bodywork and yoga will be enough, and the pain will disappear on its own.* Our bodies do not work like this. "Our issues lie in our tissues," and the issue will find a way to come to the surface! What is behind your pain? What do your body and soul want to tell you? How can you translate this body language and overcome your pain?

I found out that my pain is also related to my personal character. I am an Empath highly sensitive and highly emotionally sensitive. Based on this, I became an expert at helping highly sensitive people find their self-leadership.

Here are fifteen steps that helped me live without pain and regulate stress:

Step 1: Consult with doctors and experts to make sure nothing is medically wrong with you! You can also consult a highly qualified osteopath. All highly qualified osteopaths know when they need to send their clients to other doctors and experts for differential diagnostics. This is what I did with my clients while I was practicing osteopathy. Whenever they consulted me, I checked them holistically. When I found out something needed to be double-checked by another medical expert, I sent them to colleagues! It was never a question for me!

Step 2: Find an osteopath who can treat you holistically and is focused on craniosacral therapy/biodynamics. Please reach out to me for recommendations. There are lists of recommendations that ensure their qualifications and competency. That is very important for you to know. Some people they call themselves osteopaths and haven't studied osteopathy for five years!

Step 3: Try yoga—my favorite styles are Triyoga and Kundalini yoga.

Step 4: Meditate.

Step 5: Spend a lot of time in nature.

Step 6: Change your eating habits and figure out what energizes you. Eat regularly real, young food and focus on traffic light eating.

Step 7: Get a coach who is focused on inner work, shadow work, healing your inner/wounded child, great story work, emotional intelligence, and the shamanic path.

Step 8: Try running, swimming, and cardio training.

Step 9: Surround yourself with people who nurture you!

Step 10: Get enough sleep—and develop a regular rhythm for sleeping.

Step 11: Begin every morning intentionally and find time for thirty minutes of yoga, meditation, or setting intentions!

Step 12: Keep a journal.

Step 13: Learn to ask for help. Learn to share. Learn to take responsibility to create your reality.

Step 14: Heal your wounds and learn to manage your own life, including doing inner child work, shadow work, and ego mastery.

Step 15: Practice mindfulness.

On my professional path, I served people successfully in guiding them out of their pain and stress. As an osteopath, I witnessed many clients with physical pain. Many clients let go of pain-causing attachments that were no longer serving them. I taught my clients how to let themselves be in pain instead of fighting it. One eye-opening exercise for my clients helps them see if their lives are out of balance. They may think everything is great except for the pain. This exercise is called the wheel of life.

With the wheel of life, my clients become aware that their lives are not balanced. Some edges on the wheel of life create chaos and pain. Most of the time, the edges of their wheels are imprints from unresolved issues with work, family, health, money, childhood, or traumas. They are running on an edgy wheel instead of a balanced wheel. This causes pain. There is a disconnect between the body, mind, and soul and the truest self.

Just because you have not found a way to get out of your pain yet doesn't mean it is impossible. Don't give up! It is possible, and change is possible too. I'd like to show you the way to get there. You have put enough time and energy into all outside things. It is time to focus on you and making some changes. You will feel relieved and more relaxed. It is time to focus on you and making some changes. Very often a mental block prevents us from change and you simply don't know how…You're not alone. Many of my clients were at this stage of change. Change doesn't mean action! Change means progress and it is a dynamic, fluid process! There're different stages in a change process. I'm passionate about moving with my clients like Anna through the different stages of change from not thinking about changing a behavior, to think about it, feel it, to planing the change, taking steps toward change and finally to actually changing. Any step… is a step!

Do you want a solution that can fit into your busy life?

Welcome! You are in the right place. I'm happy to walk the path with you and next to you. You will get rid of this pain, heal your chronic pain, and manage your stress so that you can really enjoy life again and feel much better. This book will open the door and show you a way out. You will learn to see your body differently, and you will start to listen to your body differently. A new perspective may help alleviate your pain. Pain in your neck or back may have an impact on your energy level. I will reveal some client case studies and show what has changed for them and how they changed.

Here is a summary of the steps and the book structure:

Step 1: Your body is a temple. Have you ever thought about treating your body like a temple? You will get to know your body in a new way by learning about the five layers of your body. After that, you will find knowledge that can support you in getting rid of your pain.

Step 2: You will learn to really listen to your body. There are different voices in our minds and different emotions running through our bodies that cause pain. It is helpful to identify them and manage them.

Step 3: You will find new perspectives about pain and see what might be related to your pain—even if you have not thought about it before.

Step 4: It gives you insights into the energy system of the body, which is also called the chakra system. If these systems are blocked, it causes pain. You will get a greater understanding of each chakra and find exercises to work on each chakra.

Steps 5 and 6: It is all about you and your Self. These steps help with deep inner work. You will get to know your shadow side, discover and set healthy boundaries, and practice exercises to help master ourselves and nourish ourselves.

Step 7: This step gives you the experience of the power of rituals. You will try a "letting go ritual" and a "celebration ritual."

Step 8: It will make you aware of obstacles that may come after you read this book and start the process of healing and change. You will find some advice and next steps.

I've seen so many people trapped in pain, stress and losing the quality of life. I also know this feeling myself. Some days are better, and some days are really bad. It is full of ups and downs, and that is no fun at all. It is hard to enjoy meeting friends for lunch, going out for a drink, traveling, or hiking with your partner. All of these events are frustrating because of the pain. I dealt with my lower back pain, neck/shoulder pain, and emotional pain of shock trauma, abandonment and betrayal. I fought with my pain. I got out of it, and many of my clients achieved the same result.

I encourage you to face your pain and stress and take ownership! Your emotional life needs special attention. Your mental life needs special attention. Your spiritual life needs special attention and your physical body deserves special attention. The only way out is through! Your journey to vibrant health begins now.

Wherever you go, go with all your heart.
—Confucius

CHAPTER
3

YOUR BODY IS
YOUR TEMPLE

SYMPTOMS LEAD US to solutions. How do you treat your body? In the past, I expected my body to simply function in all situations. I did not take care of my body in the same way I do today. I ignored my body. I was not thinking about giving my body the right food or drinking enough water. I was also not thinking about regularly taking a break to rest, relax, or recover. I just thought I could continue going on forever. I did not listen to my body because I did not know what it meant to listen to my body. I did not know how to do it. Nobody told me or taught me. I could not sense very much of what I was feeling. My body felt numb, and my feelings were suppressed and repressed. I did not know how to express them. When I was in pain, and my body reacted with lower back pain or neck pain, I ran away from it and bypassed the pain. I treated myself very hard. Over the years, the pain became louder!

I observe the same behavior with my clients. Anna came to my session, and I asked, "What brings you to me?"

She said, "I wake up every morning with neck pain or back pain—or both. And I go to bed in pain. I can't imagine how it feels to go a day without pain. It really sucks, and I do not know what to do anymore. Nobody has helped me so far. I have no clue where this pain comes from. I also do not need to know where it comes from, but I need a quick fix to get out of it and continue with my life. My children need me, my husband needs me, my clients need me, and my team and boss need me. I have to be ready for them."

I said, "This is not going to be resolved in one or two sessions." I asked her a few more questions.

She took my comment seriously and let it sink in.

Anna treated herself and her body so hard. Like many of my clients, she was struggling in life and trying to manage her pain. However, managing and controlling almost never work!

Anna was penetrated by pain and was running in a hamster wheel. She did not know how to get out of it and break the cycle. I know how hard it is. The first step is to stop running away and face the symptom. Instead of learning how to sit with it, sit in the fire.

Anna thought everything was fine outside of her body, and she never thought there was a connection between the outside world and her inner world. I wanted her to get out of it. I wanted to guide her on her journey. This is where it starts.

It might be interesting to learn more about your body and to get to know your body more deeply. Here is a little scientific introduction that you can benefit from every day. Have you ever thought about looking at your body as a temple that deserves to be treated with a lot of compassion? Getting there will be part of your transformation.

For now, I will introduce you to the five layers of your body. When I heard about the five layers of the body the first time, I was surprised and fascinated. It opened a door to a new dimension. For the first time, I saw my body differently.

Imagine the many layers of an onion and translate this system of layers to your body. The body consists of five layers. Look at the layers from the outside to the inside:

- the physical body
- the energetic body
- the mental and emotional body
- the wisdom body
- the spiritual body

The inner layer—the spiritual body—is the seat of the soul. This is your truest Self. The core of who you are! Your essence!

The five layers of self overlap and interact. They communicate with each other and play a major role in healing and getting rid of pain. Being centered in our 5 layers of our body and emotional available create a healthy, joyful life in freedom and peace. Being not centered in your 5 layers of your body and not emotional available causes pain, discomfort, disbalance, disconnection and can cause illness.

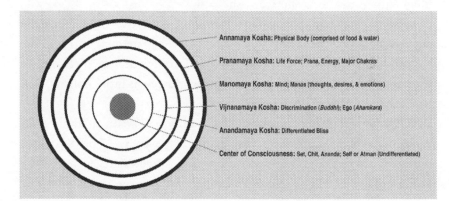

Annamaya Kosha: Physical Body (comprised of food & water)

Pranamaya Kosha: Life Force; Prana, Energy, Major Chakras

Manomaya Kosha: Mind; Manas (thoughts, desires, & emotions)

Vijnanamaya Kosha: Discrimination (*Buddhi*); Ego (*Ahamkara*)

Anandamaya Kosha: Differentiated Bliss

Center of Consciousness: Sat, Chit, Ananda; Self or Atman (Undifferentiated)

I see how things are connected between inside of us and outside of us. In Anna's first session, I notice her holistic worldview. I appreciate her openness toward seeing the things in our bodies holistically, and I do not take it for granted. She believes that everybody creates their own reality in life. That is another value I share with many of my clients. Very often, they have this belief, but they do not know how to relate it painful situations in their lives.

Anna said, "I believe I'm the creator and author of my life, but I don't know what it has to do with my pain. I didn't create my pain or wish to manifest it in reality."

I got her. Nobody consciously chooses pain. That is where I can meet Anna and many clients to help guide the hero's journey.

Coming back to your five layers, there is communication and a connection between them. That means getting or expanding the knowledge of the science of the body, developing an understanding of the energy levels that influence the body's physical functions, understanding the mind and emotions, and understanding the consciousness and spiritual/ authentic self. That may sound complicated or overwhelming, but it supports you on your journey.

All the suffering and pain we experience results in separation. The separation between the five layers is built when we do not nurture our physical bodies in healthy ways, when we ignore our emotional bodies and our thought patterns, and when we are not aware of our different energetic levels. How can you feel the difference between the layers?

Anna was confused when I explained them to her. "I have never thought about my body this way," she said.

In some worldviews, you will hear the perspective only about the body (biology) and the mind. The focus is on the material nature and the physical world. Others include the soul and consciousness, the world of the unseen, and the material world. This worldview is more holistic, and this is what Anna and I believe in.

When my clients come from the traditional medical model and checkup, they were treated as passive beings who were fixed by the doctor or drugs. They did not take responsibility and actively participate in their healing process except to deliver information about the symptoms. The symptoms lead us to the solutions that are in every one of us. With my clients, I see how things are working in life.

We are all creative, resourceful, and whole, but we often lose this belief and the connection to this natural power in us. That creates pain in us. Every human being needs to find their own perspective of the world and figure out which tools work to reduce pain and stress.

Anna and many of my other clients are taking a journey of self-exploration to the authentic self. Authentic emotions in us bring transformation and healing from pain and stress. There is no single recipe or model that works for everyone. You need to figure out what works for you.

Authenticity and emotional transparency bring us back from separation to connection. It plays a big role in the healing process. When you let go of pain and suffering, you will feel so much better. You can start to explore the five layers in your life.

THE PHYSICAL BODY AND LAYER

The physical body houses the five physical senses: seeing, tasting, eating, hearing, and smelling. It also houses our tissues and organs and the five elements. When we have an experience, it comes into our bodies through the five senses. When we see and smell something, we create a thought based on this sensation. Based on the sensation and the thought we created, we form an emotion related to it. It's a moment of decision and choice. We judge the experience as positive or negative, and we form a negative or positive thought and emotion.

The psychosomatic connection between the physical body and the mental, emotional, psychological body shows how our issues live in our tissues. Traumatic mental and emotional experiences are embedded in our physical tissues. Our issues live in our tissues.

When Anna came to me, she was not aware of how we create the emotions that can cause pain and suffering. It can come out as neck or back pain. For me, a core wound of betrayal and abandonment was sitting in my body and showing up as back pain. The work issues and marriage issues were sitting in my tissues and appearing as back pain, neck pain, and headaches.

How can you nurture your physical body? You can pay attention to food and nutrition. You can focus on real and young food and learn about traffic light eating. Traffic light eating focuses on the quality of food and tells you what green food is, what yellow food is, and what red light food is. You will learn which foods nurture you and your body and which foods weaken your immune system and trigger wear and tear, inflammation, and pain in your body.

Find exercises that are fun, and you can frequently do a combination of strengthening, cardio, and flexibility. I recommend twenty minutes of exercise every day and one cardio exercise, sport, or movement, and one calming, strengthening, flexibility, and meditative exercise, sport, or movement. Clear out on a regular basis. Clear any thoughts or toxic elements that are no longer serving your body at least twice a year. There are wonderful cleansing programs that are easy to integrate into a busy life. In the spring and fall, I do a ten-day cleansing based on Ayurveda. It is easy to integrate into a busy life.

THE SUBTLE BODY AND LAYER

The subtle body is the nonphysical psychic body that is connected to the physical body. It can be measured as electromagnetic force fields within us and around us. This field appears as spinning wheels that are called chakras. The seven chakras are located in the seven major nerve points, which are close to the spinal column. The chakras can't be seen in the physical body, but they show up in the way we think, feel, and handle situations in life. It is like the autobahn, and it runs through the body and delivers energy.

In *Eastern Body, Western Mind,* Anodea Judith, PhD, said, "Just as we see the wind through movement of the leaves and branches, the chakras can be seen by what we create around us."

You will learn about possibilities, healing, and exercises in a single chapter about chakras. It is very helpful for getting rid of pain and suffering.

THE MENTAL/EMOTIONAL BODY AND LAYER

The mental/emotional body holds our thought patterns, emotional experiences, belief patterns, and fundamental choices. It is formed by your personality type, personal history, relationship issues, family of origin issues, the story of your life, constitution, and past trauma.

We think more than fifty thousand thoughts in a day, and 80 percent of them are nonsense. When we are trapped in thought patterns and attached to emotional frequencies, we create separation within us, and that causes pain. I created a core lie and believed I was not wanted and was not lovable. I felt hurt and lonely. I also believed I was not allowed to be happy before others in my close environment—and the world—are happy.

For years, I tried to make others happy. I tried to rescue the whole world, which was totally crazy. Can you imagine how exhausting that was? It caused most of my pain. I realized what I had created in my life in a session with my coach. When it clicked, all the pressure and stress left my body. I felt a big relief and relaxation, and the pain was almost gone. You might have experienced in your culture or how you were raised to suppress your feelings. Many of us were taught to suppress them or told get over it, or here have some food, it is not a big deal....When we suppress this energy, the vibration of the emotions which includes the shadow emotions such as rage, shame, guilt, grief, fear and also joy, playfulness, happiness settle into your body system and become the tension we experience such as stress and anxiety or depression. Repressing emotions, not being centered in your 5 layers and not emotional available can operate as a kind of anesthetic and can cause pain, discomfort, imbalance, disconnection, stress, tension and illness in your body. Tension, stress, anxiety are the number one causes for illness and depression.

I invite you to explore and feel your emotions. Either express them with yourself or share your experience with someone wisely. Also, find the turn-off or calm down button so that you can have the feeling but not letting your emotions have you. While you feel your range of emotions be sure you also feel your body, your legs, and arms at the same time. Also feel your feet on the ground. And be aware of your breath. Grounding, centering and self-regulation while processing emotions is significant.

Very often we bypass our emotional body and find nice love language to talk about emotions instead really feeling them in your body and heart. I noticed that very often the language of love and light is used to not actually feel. When you bypass your emotions and choose not to feel, you might miss the huge experience of aliveness through choosing not to sit in the emotional experience and integrate them in your body and life.

It is healthy to be in relationship with all your emotions. I've to be in relation to my anger, my fear, my grief, my playfulness, my joy, fun... If I'm not in a relationship with them, if I'm denying my emotions and just use spiritual language to make it pretty I miss something. It's going hard to relate and being empathetic with someone, it's going hard to create intimacy if you're not in a relationship with your own emotions and feelings.

In my experience, it 's just freeing me to navigate consciously and establishing a healthy balance between expressing sadness, anger, hurt and cultivating lightness, playfulness and joy.

Especially for those of you who have relationships in the foreground of your attention, it is so relaxing to surrender in the experience that honoring your emotions and desires can support rather than threaten the ability to maintain and form positive, healthy, intimate relationships. I love the words from Jeanine Mancusi Co-Director of Lucid Living " Feel deeply and love powerfully."

How can you nurture your mental/emotional body? I hired a coach because I felt somebody else might be going through a process and be ahead of me. I wanted to be supported and guided through my emotional/mental process. I practiced asking for help, and I was clear that I wanted guidance and support.

What is part of this process? Inner work, shadow work, healing the inner child, awakening the nurturing parent in us, building relationship skills, building communication skills, building healthy boundaries, processing emotions, and learning to understand them. Real change is an emotional process, and I highly recommend asking for help!

THE WISDOM BODY AND LAYER

The higher mind is in the third eye, which is centered between the eyebrows. It is also called the inner eye. It is connected to the higher mind and has the capacity to develop our inner witness of consciousness, our inner teacher, and our inner healer.

How can you nurture the wisdom body? Learn to stabilize and strengthen the mind by slicing away thoughts and beliefs that no longer serve you. Develop mindfulness and observe the thought patterns and the emotional forms that result from it. Don't be stuck with it—and cultivate healthy action.

With Anna and many other clients, we practiced a different kind of meditation. Anna was trapped in a thought pattern that she was not good enough. She was striving to please everybody. That caused her pain and restlessness. Through meditation, she learned to activate the inner voice of her observer, and she practiced detachment.

THE SPIRITUAL BODY AND LAYER

The spiritual body is the spirit and the soul. In the core of the soul is the essence or the center of consciousness and self. The spirit and soul are essence, life force, and life energy. It is who we are without masks in our entire purification, innocence, and vulnerability. This part of us cocreates with the unseen. States of peak experiences in life are part of our core essence. It contains passion, boundless love, enthusiasm, bliss, joy, peace, creativity, and sexual ecstasy. It is the part of us that shines bright like a star, the moon, or the sun. Many of us have been taught not to shine too brightly, but it is our birthright to shine as fully in the world as we can.

We can nurture the spiritual body by exploring the spiritual body, surrounding ourselves with like-minded people, studying, self-exploring, meditating, and practicing shamanic journeying.

In spiritual psychology, we ask, "Who am I?" I hope you have a new understanding of your body systems, how the layers are interconnected, and each layer's function. When I first heard about all the pieces, it was fascinating and overwhelming. I needed to digest each step. In time, I learned to integrate each layer, build my own relationship, and connect with each of the five bodies.

It has made a big difference in my life. I let go of the pain and engaged in self-exploration, healing, change, and transformation from the inside out and the outside in. The most impactful experience was my growing understanding of the mental/emotional body and doing my inner work and shadow work. I still do inner work and shadow work. It will never end, and I believe that life is our curriculum.

Seeing the body in five layers helps you understand how to work through the five layers that cover your deepest core essence, your truest self, and your soul. It is learning how to optimize your physical body, your energetic body, and your emotional/mental body. It is about accessing more and more of your core self. It is about going home to your truest self.

How do you balance and restore your body systems with all five layers? Stay tuned and find out more in the next chapters.

Connecting and Nurturing Each of the Five Layers

Buddha said, "The body is our vehicle for awakening—treat it with great care."

We have to take care of all five layers so that our wisdom and spiritual bodies can flourish. The physical body must be properly nourished and exercised to provide a strong spirit to manifest the heart's desires. The mental body has to be clear and at peace with itself. The emotional body has to be elevated with emotions like joy, gratitude, and authentic self-love. How do we pay attention to each layer?

THE PHYSICAL BODY AND LAYER

Balanced nutrition connects the physical body. Not every physical body is the same! Each body is different. We are all different. There is a lot of great nutritional advice, but people have different bodies. Not all nutritional needs, plans, and bodies are equal. Our bodies are always changing, and what worked for us in the past may not necessarily be good or effective for us now. How do we work around this? Tune in to your body's wisdom and understand its language. It has all the answers you are looking for. I educate and motivate my clients to learn all about the quality of food, traffic light eating, and eating real and young food. They learn the secrets about their individual retirement accounts for health and much more. Proper nutrition is very important because poor nutrition is directly related to illness and inflammation that may cause pain and stress in our bodies. Here are just a few of the problems people who have poor nutrition may experience. Obesity or being overweight, having low self-esteem, Typ 2 diabetes, being sick with an illness like colds and flu more often, having learning difficulties or trouble concentrating, kids with poor nutrition often have behavior problems and both adults and kids have trouble concentrating.

Pediatricians are very concerned about the childhood obesity trends because for the first time in history a child's parents will likely live more years than their own children.

When I heard about this new trend I was shocked and my heart cramps because I feel so sad about this development and I so want it different for all of us.

Real food has an impact on the cellular level. Cells grow better that eat better and the genetic reproduction is better. Real food makes you feel better and gives you more sustainable energy. It is about finding the balance between real food and junk food.

Cleansing on a regular basis connects your body. Once or twice a year, clean and detox the GI tract, liver, blood, and lymphatic system.

Your health is a pure reflection of how good your digestion is. It all starts with your digestive system. Your gut, consisting of your small and large intestine, harbors 75 percent of your immunity, makes critical vitamins, and controls hormones, including most serotonin production, which is needed for being happy and joyful. If your gut is happy, you will be happy. You will feel well rested after a good night's sleep, have energy all day, and enjoy the way you feel inside.

Exercise and movement connects the physical body. Don't find excuses. Never say you don't have time. That excuse means your body and your self aren't important to you. I recommend twenty minutes every day. Make movements your priority and your medicine. We spend time and money on so many other things, but body movement should be a priority. Movements provide physical and emotional well-being. Personalize your program and find movements that are fun for you. Make sure that you get in all three types of exercise: strength building exercises for your muscles and bones, cardio, and stretching.

Make it fun, start low and go slow.

THE SUBTLE BODY AND LAYER

Yoga and breathing techniques connect the energetic body. Osteopathic medicine, especially craniosacral therapy, biodynamic, and acupuncture help balance this layer. Working with your chakras with affirmations, essential oils, and special yoga exercises stimulates and awakens your energetic body.

THE MENTAL/EMOTIONAL BODY AND LAYER

For the emotional/mental body and layer, be authentic with your emotions, thoughts, and beliefs. Connect with your emotions and feel your feelings. Step into your truest self. Your thoughts, feelings, beliefs, decisions, and choices create your reality.

Look for a mind-set coach or a great story coach who offers process-oriented psychology, shamanic journey, yoga, mindfulness work, shadow work, or inner child work. These methods connect you with your emotional/mental body, and I highly recommend taking at least a few sessions. An expert can hold the space with warmth and trust so you can explore and emotions and thoughts you may be trapped in or stuck with. You will learn to set the foundation and find the tools for your life. From there, you can move forward on your own. You will be empowered with your new tools.

THE WISDOM BODY AND LAYER

Meditation can connect you to your wisdom body. Being in and with nature can connect you to your wisdom and your inner knowing. I offer beautiful meditations such as stress reduction-meditation, body-scan meditation, and breathing meditation. Reach out and ask for instruction.

THE SPIRITUAL BODY AND LAYER

Find like-minded people and circles and hang around with them to nurture the spiritual body. Study meditation, learn rituals, and have experiences with the divine/the universe/your higher self/God—you name it as you like. Learn and practice shamanic journeying.

DISCONNECTING THE FIVE LAYERS

1. Physical Body: Bad habits include eating junk food, drinking too much alcohol, sitting all the time, not moving the body at all, and being a couch potato.
2. Subtle Body: Pay attention to your breath and focus on your breath, especially in times of change, transition, or stress. Make little changes such as changing from sitting to standing. Many people hold their breath, which interrupts the flow in your body. The breath gives life. Eating old, unhealthy food on a regularly basis lowers the energy and defeats the energetic body.
3. Mental/Emotional Body: Don't be trapped in negative thought patterns and beliefs. Don't resist feeling your feelings. Those

behaviors create tension and constriction in the body and mind, causing pain and draining life energy.

4. Wisdom Body: Enjoy meditation, nature, rituals, and other practices that guide you deeper into You.
5. Spiritual Body: Co-dependency and toxic relationships. The unawareness and avoidance of exploring your true Self. The false believe in your false self and inner critic.

Here's a fun way to become more aware of the single layers:

Which activity matches which body?

1. meditation
2. hummus with pita
3. setting healthy boundaries
4. gratitude jar
5. dancing
6. yoga
7. orange essential oil
8. massage
9. sweat lodge
10. shamanic rituals

Answers:

1. balances the wisdom body, spiritual body, and mental/emotional body
2. balances the physical body
3. balances the mental/emotional body
4. balances the energetic body (gratitude generates high energy) and mental/emotional body
5. balances the physical body
6. balances all five bodies
7. balances the energetic body
8. balances the physical body
9. balances all five bodies
10. balances the wisdom and spiritual body mostly

CHAPTER
4

LISTENING TO
YOUR BODY

IN THIS CHAPTER, I want to focus on your pain.
It took me a while to learn what to do with my pain after I got the green light from the medical world that I was healthy. I was so focused on traditional ways before I thought about trying out new ideas and unconventional medical techniques. It took me a while to be open and open myself to walk the path differently. It was the same for Anna with her non-stoppable neck and back pain.

She said, "Which path should I follow? I feel like I'm on a dead-end street. I can turn right or left. Turning right means following the traditional medical path, and turning left means trying something new and following the alternative medical path."

Anna decided to follow the alternative medical path, and that was the day I met her in my practice. That was the beginning of her new journey toward get rid of the pain. I told her to focus on following the alternative path, and I advised her to combine it if needed with the traditional medical path. I'm a big advocate of mixing both for the sake of healing and managing pain and stress.

When Anna told me about her pain, I started listening to her on different levels and between the lines. I introduced her to the different approach I'm using. I was primarily coaching her and consulting holistically, but I sometimes combine it with osteopathy or yoga and meditation. She was open to exploring a new way. She only wanted to get rid of the pain. She was not aware that her daily life issues were sitting in the tissues of her neck and back and causing endless pain. She was not aware of her five layers.

In one of our first sessions, I used the wheel of life exercise. I have used it with many of my clients at the beginning of their journeys with me. It considers each area of your life and makes you aware of what is off balance. It is useful when life has gotten out of balance.

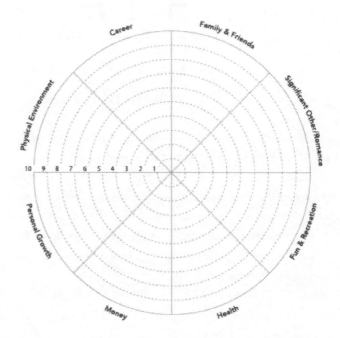

When life is busy—or all your energy is focused on a special project or area of your life—it's easy to find yourself off balance and not paying enough attention to important areas of your life. While you're focusing on getting things done, taking this too far can lead to frustration, intense stress, and pain. That's when it's time to take an eagle view and bring things back into balance.

The wheel of life is powerful because it gives you a vivid visual representation of the way your life is currently going and compares it with the way you'd ideally like it to be. It is called the wheel of life because each area of your life is mapped on a circle, like the spokes of a wheel. The concept was originally created by Paul J. Meyer, founder of

Success Motivation Institute, Inc. You can score each section from one to ten. One is the lowest score, and ten is the highest score you can give. When you do the exercise, you will see where you are in your life by making a cross on the number in each section. At the end, you can connect all the crosses and see how balanced or unbalanced your wheel is.

The circle represents your life and the whole of you. The spokes show the aspects of your life: family, business, health, and money. The idea is to make you aware of these aspects, to see where you are in your life, and to determine if there are significant issues you've been neglecting or giving away. Those issues show up in your tissues as pain.

Anna said, "I can't ignore my pain anymore. It has become so intense. I really hope to resolve it here. What is this wheel about? What does it have to do with my case?"

The purpose of the wheel is to make you aware and wake you up to see what you need when life is out of balance. Many of my clients are not aware that their lives are out of balance. They are convinced that everything in life is great except for the pain. It was the same way for me. They do not make the correlation between pain and being out of balance. This is the first secret and key. Your pain is saying, "Stop ignoring me. Listen to me. Your life is out of balance!" You can see the pain as a big stop sign and wake-up call.

The wheel shows us when all our attention and energy are put into work or family and when we are ignoring our health, need for joy, abundance, fun, and creativity, and many of the juicy pieces of life. When one aspect of life is getting much more attention than the other ones, the wheel becomes wobbly and eventually crashes.

The goal is to get back to balance and restore our system to make it whole. And by wholeness I mean health! *Whole* is the origin of *health*, but it means more than the health of the physical body. It means health and the balance between all five layers. It addresses the balance between the physical body, mental/emotional, energetic, spirit and wisdom/mind-body.

The wheel of life is an eye-opener for most of my clients. Anna was stunned and scared to see that she put too much energy into her family, marriage, and work. She was striving to be the best mom, the best wife, and the best manager without considering how it looked to be her best self. She was in the hamster wheel of giving and giving and giving to others, and she totally forgot how to give to herself or receive. She forgot to set healthy boundaries and say no to things she didn't like to do. She did them because of obligation.

Does that sound familiar to you? So many of my clients are striving in life and end up being stressed out, in pain, exhausted, restless, depressed, anxious, and afraid.

The wheel of life lets you pause, look at your life, check in on where you are in the present moment, and listen to your body and the voice of pain.

I invite you to pause, take a deep breath, and listen to your body and feelings. Is the message of your pain saying anything? How many times have you ignored your pain, whether emotionally or physically? How many times have you repressed emotional and physical pain by taking painkillers or other things to numb you or distract you from pain? How many times have you avoided your feelings and emotions by running away or escaping? How many times have you calmed the symptoms instead of seeking the roots?

When we feel pain, we tend to forget it is the way the body lets us know it needs attention. The symptoms can inform us. Feelings can inform us. For instance, a sore throat can tell us to rest our voices or give us the hint of expressing what's cooking by voicing it. Headaches can be a sign of stress or hunger. All too often, we ignore our feelings, put them aside, or avoid dealing with them. In the same way, we often avoid or ignore body pain and symptoms. If we avoid dealing with them, we'll contain them in our bodies and minds. That is when pain, anxiety, depression, and other health issues come up. All those signals are wake-up calls to pay attention to the body-mind-soul system. If we ignore the messages, the condition could become worse. There is a disconnection between our minds and bodies.

Emotional pain also gives us also valuable messages about the psyche and soul. It's a sign that we've been affected by something that needs awareness. We need to focus on the inner world. Sitting in the waves of feelings, no matter how scary they might be, is the best thing we can do for ourselves and trusting the power of the self-healing forces within us. Our feelings and emotions just want to be seen, heard, and felt. Sometimes we make it too complicated and try to analyze it or find the solutions. The deeper purpose of our feelings and emotions is to transform that inner world, opening the space for more feelings, giving the opportunity to grow, and following the river of flow. If we listen to the emotional and physical pain/symptoms, we'll know what to do and how to heal ourselves.

It's part of human nature to avoid listening to painful symptoms, feelings, and emotions. We live in a culture that does not support the awareness of emotions, feelings, and pain. I encourage you to open up and take a moment to listen to the valuable message of the pain or symptoms—either physical or emotional—and sit with your feelings before repressing or numbing them. Many of my clients avoid feeling or are afraid to feel. They protect themselves by controlling their feelings and create a wall of protection around them. That makes it difficult to reach them. Anna built a wall around her and kept it so strongly that her neck and back started to hurt. When she began to explore her emotional pain, the wall melted—and the pain lessened.

All we need to do is give the process permission by leaning in, opening up, and receiving the messages from the feelings, emotions, and pain. Feeling the hurt or the unpleasant feelings does not have to be frightening. It is not always fun to feel the painful feelings, and it is more comfortable to feel pleasant, happy feelings, but we do not need to avoid them. They are just feelings, and we can surrender to them, feel them, and then go on. Emotional pain does not have to confuse us. We can sit in the fire, sit still, feel the pain, figure out if there is something we need to take care of ourselves, and move on in life. We can begin to share our feelings with others. That brings relief and healing to us and to them because if you take the lead on it and share first, you allow others to do the same.

When we first sit in the fire and do not know how to express our feelings, it might be more useful, valuable, and easier to start exploring with a coach. An experienced coach guided me through the process. It is a beautiful experience to share and to be seen and heard by somebody! It is a life-changing process! Real change is an emotional process! This is happening with many of my clients.

Surrendering to our feelings—even the emotionally painful ones—and being open and vulnerable enough to feel the feelings is a powerful act of taking responsibility for all our feelings. I always feel so grateful when my clients are brave enough to step out of their comfort zones and reach the places of deepest vulnerability. They show up as if they are completely naked. Holding the space and witnessing this process is very sacred! The process of emotional authenticity and transparency makes them feel free of pain, stress, and pressure.

After discovering Anna's wheel of life, we stepped into the exploration of her mental/emotional body. One tool that is very impactful is called the tiers of emotions. It shows a range of twenty-one emotional frequencies that are living naturally within us. It is a great tool to make these frequencies aware of us, wake up hidden parts of us, and integrate them again.

Many of my clients have learned to listen to their bodies on a deeper level and identify their emotional frequencies. As you can see in the image below, some emotions create constriction in us and some create expansion. A few are in the category of generating imprisoning energy, and a couple are in the field of transitioning energy. You can explore your feelings and get to know yourself better by differentiating these feelings in coaching. When I worked with Anna, we explored her whole range of emotions. It was very freeing for her.

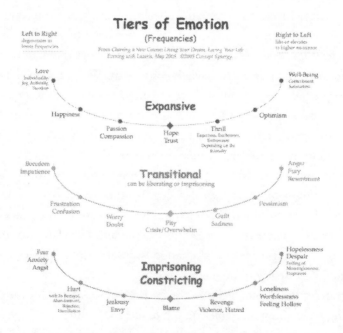

Tiers of Emotion by Lazaris

Start Working with Your Emotions

Begin to identify and express the emotions you are feeling. Which emotions take up the most space in your frequencies of emotions? Are you addicted to any particular emotions that have become your default? There's no right or wrong. All emotions are allowed.

In addition to the emotional part, we started to listen to Anna's mental body and to all the voices that are talking to her. A huge voice is a critical voice that always wants to judge her and tell her how bad she is, that she's not good enough, unwanted, and unloved.

I remember how hard it was for me to learn to differentiate between the voices within me. I see it with many of my clients. It takes a while to notice which voice is talking inside myself and taking the lead. Is it the critical voice with limiting thoughts and belief patterns? Is it the criticized inner child? Is it the voice that comes from a deeply heartfelt, open, vulnerable, nurturing place? These voices are our inner critics and nurturing parent voices.

When we are in pain, we lose this connection and access to the nurturing piece in us. Most of my clients can hear their critical, self-sabotaging voice very clearly and loudly, and the nurturing voice is very often in the background and very quiet.

The self-sabotaging mind talk creates separation from wisdom and the spiritual body. Remember the five layers. When we are trapped and attached in this mental/emotional layer and guided by limiting thought patterns and depressing feelings, it is hard to move forward, get to the next layers, and access the most authentic self and the soul. It almost holds us back, and we spiral down energetically. It keeps us away from being fluid and flexible, and it keeps us trapped in one layer. It keeps us trapped in one box, which causes pain and suffering.

When I went with Anna into the deeper levels in her process of self-exploration, I gave her homework to practice body scan exercises every day and take time out for herself on a regular basis. Body scan meditation, pain meditation, and mindful eating kept her training muscles she explored and became aware of in our sessions.

We can start living the new awareness by integrating it into our daily lives and walking new paths. Most of my clients are committed to it and recognize the benefits of their new knowledge. It helps their dream come true of getting rid of the pain on a long-term basis.

For Anna and many of my clients, four keys were very supportive after they stepped into the deeper levels of self-exploration and listening to the body:

- Key 1: Mindfulness: building awareness of the body, feelings, and thoughts.
- Key 2: Understanding: Changing your view and developing an understanding of the nature of things.
- Key 3: Thoughts: Avoiding thoughts of attachment, hatred, and harmful intention and correcting the intention.
- Key 4: Words: Your words have weight and can either hurt or empower. Be aware of the words you're choosing. Gossip, senseless, harsh speech, and lying can create harm.

Anna wrote these keys on a Post-It and stuck it on the mirror in the bathroom to be reminded every day.

She said, "On this journey of coaching, I learned very impressively and sustainably how much wisdom is in the body and how much the body is talking/whispering nonverbally—and you only need to listen!"

If we can move toward the pain—rather than pushing it away—and shift the awareness around it, we might be surprised by what we find. Most of my clients learned that what you resist persists.

BODY SCAN MEDITATION

The body scan helps us ground our attention and arrive in our bodies. Since the body is always in the present moment, when we are aware of our bodies, we are automatically aware of the present moment—the here and now.

The body scan meditation can be done sitting up or lying down. It is a type of meditation that uses the sensations in the body as attention.

- Take a comfortable and relaxed position, either sitting or lying down, and close your eyes.
- Take a moment to go inward and recall your motivation for meditating. You can imagine how you want to feel in the future or how you want to be in relation to others.
- Bring your attention to your sensations in your body, starting with the tips of your toes. How do your toes feel? Notice the sensation in your toes. How do you know that your toes are there if you can't see them?
- Move up in your body and graduate your awareness from your feet to your lower legs, upper legs, hips, stomach, torso, lower/middle/upper back, shoulders, arms, hands, neck, head, and face. Bring the same curiosity and nonjudgmental attention to each part of your body and discover the sensations. Pause frequently along the way to just notice the sensations that are showing up in the present moment.
- Take a few moments to rest in awareness of all the sensations in your body as a whole and observe your breathing. Silently observe your sensations and breathing before you open your eyes.
- When you open your eyes, look around the room and notice what is around you. You can thank your body and conclude the body scan meditation session.

CHAPTER
5

PAIN AND HIGHLY EMOTIONALLY SENSITIVITY

ANNA IS HIGHLY sensitive, highly emotionally sensitive, and an empath. Over the years, I have observed a deep connection between pain and highly sensitive people (HSP), highly emotionally people, and empaths. Anna's lower back pain and neck pain became chronic, which was an expression of her personal character and HSP. The pain was a sign to stop and change her life.

When I was in pain, a book crossed my path. It was a book about HSP, and it was so precious for me. I saw myself in it, and I saw the connection between my pain, this personal gift, and vulnerability. It was an additional puzzle that helped me understand myself better. That was a key element in the healing process of Anna, many other clients, and myself.

What is high sensitivity? The term high sensitivity (HS) or highly sensitive person was characterized in the 1990s by American psychologist and psychotherapist Dr. Elaine N. Aron. It is a personal characteristic expressed by increased sensitivity and perception. Furthermore, perceived information is experienced significantly more intensely.

It is assumed that 15–20 percent of the population are highly sensitive. Every fifth person in Germany has an increased sensitivity, which is seen as a personal characteristic and not as a disease or disorder. Also, 20 percent of children are highly sensitive. Dr. Elaine Aron considers this an evolutionary development.

HSP personal characteristics include:

- vivid imagination
- tendency to perfectionism
- increased sensitivity to injustice and mistakes
- explicitly strong intuition
- thinking in larger contexts
- strong tendency to question things
- search for meaning
- intensive experiencing and perception
- increased diligence in acting
- increased empathy
- increased suggestibility by feelings of others
- self-worth problems due to experiences of rejection
- feeling different
- increased risk for anxiety disorders, depression, burnout, traumatic stress disorders, and psychosomatic symptoms due to inner burnout

Highly sensitive people have finer perception and more accurate perception because of their more sensitive nervous systems and less filter in their system of perception. This causes overstimulation of the body, mind, and soul system faster than usual due to fewer filters of perception. There's a higher perception of noises, a higher sensitivity to the quality of the air or weather in general, a very fine perception of optical irritations and impressions, and a more intense perception of inner emotional worlds. They experience their inner worlds in richer and more detailed ways. Their intuition is very high. Very often, they are moved and touched by music, art, and nature.

They tend to be overstimulated faster than other people. For this reason, it is important to get to know oneself well as an HSP and to become aware of your gift and vulnerability at the same time to step fully into your potential without being exhausted by high sensations and perceptions and without containing it all in pain. In some situations, one HSP might feel deeply hurt because he or she is so sensitive, open, and permeable.

As an HSP, you might remember responses you've received when you reacted to something very sensitive, and people told you not to be so sensitive. You might feel like something is weird when you enter a room. That kind of perception is very common. It is helpful to learn about the characteristics of an HSP and how you can take care of yourself to build a loving relationship with yourself and with others. In many situations, it might be helpful to know more about your potential as a highly sensitive person:

- work
- health
- intimate relationships, love, and romance
- work-life-balance and fulfilment in life
- leadership

HSPs tend to play the victim role instead of being leaders and owning this privilege and unique gift. For many of my clients, high sensitivity and being highly emotional and empathetic is a part of their lives; they often run out of balance. It shows up in chronic pain, stress, exhaustion, restlessness, sleep disorders, depression, anxiety, and burnout. Their wheel of life is wobbly!

The following steps for self-care apply to everyone, but for HSPs, they are particularly helpful. My HSP clients have benefited a lot from these steps, which helped them live without pain. I highly recommend to practice grounding, self-regulation and centering every day. Practice, practice, practice !

- Visit nature regularly to clean your system, gain clarity, reconnect with yourself, and become centered and refreshed.
- Drink healthy juices and smoothies. Your body needs healthy food to support your subtle body and stay balanced because it is very sensitive to food.
- Meditate and pay attention to your inner peace. Listen to it what is going on inside you. What is alive? How does it feel? Meditation cleanses, empowers, and focuses on what is essential in life.
- Be well and stable in your body to keep your energy household stable. The more one is centered, the more energy one has, and the tendency to be overstimulated shrinks.

- Eat healthy, nurturing food (including dark chocolate in reasonable proportions)
- Move, try stress-reducing breathing meditation, get enough sleep every night, try yoga, or walk, hike, or spend time in nature.
- Bring your emotions into balance. The more you're feeling your feelings, the more you are emotionally available and centered.
- Sometimes it is enough to put one hand on your heart and breathe into your heart.

These four steps for mindfulness are also good for slowing down and calming down before taking the next step:

- pause
- breathe
- soften
- feel

And then take the next step of action.

Sports and movement bring your energy into flow, reduce stress hormones, and activates the body's circulation and digestive systems. Fresh outdoor air can get into all your cells and renew your body, and all stalled air can be let go off. It activates your cells, makes your body feel alive, and fills you with energy.

Connecting with your creative parts balances you, relaxes you, and slows down your body, mind, and soul system. The creative part of the brain is the right side. The left side of the body is connected to the right side of the brain.

Here's an easy and fun exercise to stimulate the right, creative side of your brain. Most people brush their teeth with their right hand. Just turn around and break your habit by brushing your teeth with your left hand. This stimulates and trains the right side of your brain and your creative side.

Another routine you can create in your daily life is journaling every morning. What does it mean? Try writing three pages of stream of consciousness. Just write anything that is coming out without pausing or thinking. Keep the flow of writing even if you write "I don't know what I should write" or "blah, blah, blah." Just write three pages. It is not supposed to sound great or make sense. It is not about right and wrong. It is only about connecting you with your creative side, and writing is meant as creative recovery. Why journaling? Morning journaling on a regular basis will get you to the other side of your fears, negativity, victimhood, and moods. It will soothe the critical voice inside and empower the conscious creator. Benefits of journaling: stress reduction, personal growth, healing, knowing yourself and truth better, captures your life story, enhances intuition and creativity.

For Anna, it was crucial, especially when she became aware of her HSP. She learned to take care of herself, cultivate a healthy relationship with herself, balance her body, mind, and soul system, and clear her energy household. Self-care is significant for all of us, and all my clients need self-care awareness and mindfulness. I emphasize it here for HSP because it is twice as essential to be aware of to get rid of the pain.

To find out more about HSP or empaths or if you are categorized as HSP, you can reach out to me. HSP has nothing to do with being an introvert. HSP and introversion or extroversion can overlap. They are two different shoes. This information has confused some of my clients.

If you're interested in learning more exercises or getting more instructions and tools, email me at ab@annabelle-breuer.com. I'd love to talk to you.

CHAPTER
6

NEW PERSPECTIVES

WHEN ANNA CALLED me for her first coaching session, she had no perspective. She was stuck and trapped in her neck and back pain. It was a dead-end street for her. She complained and said, "I have no hope anymore. I'm desperate, and nobody can help me."

"Well, you can help yourself out," I said.

The next time she consulted me, she opened her heart to let me see more into her and her life. She was not talking only about the pain and where it hurt. She needed to get rid of it as soon as possible so that she could go back to her daily life. She started sharing more about her life. "My pain is getting worse every day. Almost every night, I wake up and can't find a pain-free position. I don't know how to sit at my desk in the office or in team meetings. The coaching sessions with my clients are not exciting anymore. Playing with my children is a disaster, and my sexual life with my husband is also affected. I'm not myself anymore. I can't participate in my daily life activities as I'm used to doing."

I was very moved when she opened her heart, and I knew how she was feeling. I invited her to dive deeper into the aspects of her wheel of life, which we scored in her first session. Three aspects of her life were out of balance and very wobbly: her marriage, her relationship with her boss and her team, and her health.

I said, "Anna, which issue do you want to focus on? Where do you feel you need to shine a spotlight in our session today?"

She said, "My pain is driving me nuts. Maybe I only need to do more exercises, and then it will disappear on its own—and everything will be fine."

I said, "Wait a moment, Anna. I feel like you want to escape here right now to avoid shining a spotlight on an important issue in your life that seems to be not working anymore."

Many of my clients try to escape when it comes to the point of feeling emotions or moving into uncomfortable issues.

Anna broke down in tears. "I'm afraid. My marriage is a tragedy. My husband was complaining about our sex life for a long time and put me under so much pressure. After our children were born, the relationship between my husband and me changed. It is not like it was. He cheated on me. I'm deeply hurt, and I feel numb and speechless. I feel like I want to forgive him, but it's difficult to build trust again. I don't know why he is doing this to me. Am I'm not good enough for him? I don't get any quiet moments anymore. Every day, my mind is spinning around what is he doing. Will he meet another woman? I have not told anybody what is going on in our marriage. I kept it as a secret until now." When she shared it in our session, the secret was unlocked, the silence was broken, and the energy of her pain was unleashed.

Anna was relieved to share what had been cooking in her mind for so long. She was giving herself permission to share her feelings. Her mind and her self-talk were avoiding the pain. When she listened to herself, her inner voice said, "Don't pay too much attention to this problem. With time, the wound will heal. Just move on in life and get over it. Your kids need you, and you need to be focused at work. Do not think too much about it. Even though it hurts, focus on the important things in life. It is not worth it, and the pain and disappointment will disappear in time. But I love my husband, and I thought he was the love of my life. How could this happen?"

These inner voices are so familiar, and I notice this phenomenon with so many clients. The inner critic is controlling, self-sabotaging, and judging. It says, "Don't do this. Do that." It tries to keep us away from healing and pushes us to bypass the pain. Often these voices are minimizing things that had a big impact on us and our lives.

I said, "These crazy voices are normal! Nothing is wrong with you, Anna. The way to process them is not to ignore them. It is making them aware by listening to them, learning to understand them, and identifying them."

Try to identify your nurturing inner parent voice and your critical inner parent voice. We can use certain phrases to train our inner nurturing parent voice. It helps you be mindful about your thoughts. Good inner parent messages are helpful for becoming more mindful with your emotional body. Use them as secret weapon in your pocket. Becoming more mindful and emotionally intelligent is taking responsibility for your emotional life, and it helps us learn to parent ourselves. We become emotionally free, authentic, autonomous, and compassionate toward ourselves and others.

The Nurturing Inner Parent Voice (Good Parent Voice)

- I hear you, I see you, and I love you.
- I'll take care of you.
- You can trust me.
- Sometimes I'll tell you no, and it's because I love you.
- I will set limits.
- I am proud of you.
- I give you permission to be a sexual being.
- I have confidence in you.
- If you fall down, I will pick you up.
- I give you permission to love and enjoy your sexuality with a partner of your choice and not lose me.
- I accept and cherish you.
- You don't have to be alone anymore.
- You can trust your inner voice.
- You don't have to be afraid anymore.
- You are beautiful and handsome.

The Critical Inner Parent Voice

- It is critical, judgmental, and controlling.
- It puts you down.
- It is conditional.
- It tells you you're wrong and don't matter.
- It doesn't care about your emotions, desires, wishes, and needs.
- It is the voice of perfectionism.
- It is the voice that makes decisions without checking in the voice of the inner child (intuition).
- It is the voice that ignores.
- I don't like you.
- You are not good enough.
- You are too sensitive.
- You are too emotional.
- Don't take it so seriously—it's not worse.
- You will get a reward if you do this and that.
- You are too much.
- You are too loud.
- You are talking too much. Be silent when adults are talking.
- Your wishes and desires don't matter.
- You don't matter.
- Be perfect and strong.
- Be good and behave yourself.
- Don't be who you are because that isn't good enough.
- Don't be egoistic, don't put yourself on number one, and be modest.
- Hold back. Don't tell us what you want or need.
- Don't say no, don't set boundaries, and don't take care of yourself.
- Always take care of others before you take care of yourself.
- Don't be silly or have fun.
- Don't enjoy life.
- Don't be open, honest, or direct. Instead, manipulate.
- Don't come too close to others because you make yourself vulnerable.

- Don't disturb the system by initiating growth and change.
- Always show a smiling face—no matter how you feel or what you have to do.
- Guess what others need and want—and expect the same from others

Very often, they are related to a wound that has not healed or has been ignored. The messages become conscious and open. Once you understand them, you can stop their influence and stop sabotaging your life. The messages often represent people, experiences, issues, and places in the past and present that affect your life. Anna's pain was the door to listening to her body and the messages of her voices. The voice was the pain held back in her body. The issue in Anna's marriage lived in her tissues, and her neck and back pain were expressing the screams of her soul. She opened the door courageously and listened to them—and her beautiful side and strength came out.

While we were exploring her marriage issue, another deep hurt in her life came on the surface. "I was beaten by my father in my youth twice." She was so calm when she started sharing, but a lot of anger was coming out. I held her with compassion as this huge moment came out of its hidden corner. That was all the pain she carried in her shoulders, neck, and back.

When a wound is arrested or a feeling is repressed, especially anger and hurt, a person grows up with an angry wound. You may have heard about the inner child. This can be a wound from childhood. If it is still working in us, it will contaminate the person's adult life and behavior.

This neglected, abandoned, wounded inner child of the past is the major source of human distress, and it causes a lot of pain in the world. I know how painful these moments of coming out are, and my clients have resources to heal their pain. They can activate the inner healer to let go of pain, transform their pain, and get back to daily life in a new way or with a new identity.

I encourage my clients to heal their wounds by doing inner work. I appreciate my clients who dare to be honest with themselves and stop betraying themselves. They face their issues and listen to their bodies and the screams of their souls. Our bodies are so intelligent, and they have so much wisdom. They tell us the truth about pain.

A lot of my clients have lost their feelings and the connections to their bodies' wisdom, and the pain is one channel for them to reconnect with their bodies, minds, and souls. Channels are how we perceive and experience. These channels can be body movement, relationship, dream/ vision, listening/hearing, and/or the world as a channel. Anna perceived and experienced the channel of relationship and the body channel. These occurrences are communicating through a relationship or are felt in a relationship. Her pain was an expression and a signal that took the communication through her body and in her relationship with her husband. It was related to the relationship with her father, her boss, and her team members, but that came out later in her coaching process. The pain communicates through systems such as the family of origin, marriage, or work. It shows up very often in our bodies. The issue of power and abuse of power is related to this.

My body showed me clearly through pain, tension, and pressure that something was not okay. My body and the screams of my soul showed me that I needed to change the course of my life. I needed to change it. Nobody could do it for me. It took me a while, but I learned to translate this language of my body and take action.

There is another channel that is called the world. For many of my clients, especially for the highly sensitive people and empaths, this is the channel where they feel world events. After the election in the United States in 2016, cultural fears and worldwide fears surfaced. Some of my clients reacted with headaches, and this is an example of something in the world working through us or within us.

Abuse of power in any relationships—marriage, partnership, work relationships, or systems—people often feel it in their bodies. They feel like victims and are put into boxes of humiliation and inferiority. How do we feel when we have been victimized? Powerless, helpless, trapped, frustrated, and enraged.

Anna felt powerlessness and trapped in a role as the victim with her husband and her father. She said, "Why is this happening to me? Why do they do this to me? I need somebody who can rescue me. I don't know how I can move forward or get out of this prison. I'm aware that my pain, tension, restlessness, and sleep disorder have something to do with my relationship with my husband, but I don't know what to do. I don't know what I want. I can't see the light at the end of the tunnel."

I could hear the voice of the victim as she told this story. She had lost her identity and was not in touch with her feelings, needs, and desires.

Anna started learning to identify when she was feeling victimized and why she was feeling victimized. We all have our individual victim stories going on in our lives next to our overcoming stories and great stories. We can learn to identify the different voices in these stories and we can become aware of them, own them, and change them. This happens when we realize what it is going on and why it is happening in our lives.

In Anna's recovery process, she became aware of what was happening in her life and understood more and more why it was happening. She started owning her power, learning to take care of herself, and removing herself as a victim. By owning our power, we become aware that we are victimizing ourselves. Sometimes we realize that we are victimized by another's behavior and need to set healthy boundaries to take care of ourselves.

Anna stepped out of her victim role, and she was able to open her wall of protection and numbness to feel the range of her emotions. A lot of anger, sadness, rejection, and abandonment were contained in her pain. We spent time feeling her pain and the emotions that came out of it. We have twenty-one emotions running through our bodies. With lots of compassion, she started recognizing herself differently and acknowledging her emotions. She was sitting with her feelings and allowing her emotions to be. She was slowing down and getting a glimpse of her soul wherever she was in her phase of development. It was only about being with Anna in this exploration.

In today's world, especially with such fast development of technology, we tend to check things off our to-do lists and spend more time doing, doing, doing, and we forget our beautiful side of just being.

Anna was sometimes tired after a coaching session.

"This is normal," I said. "You did amazing inner work. Your body is reacting to it and letting go of toxins and burned inner blockades. Nurture your body, drink warm water as much as possible to support your body in this process, and take an Epsom bath as often as you want for at least thirty minutes. Epsom salt helps us detox. It is good for support when we release a lot through processing. Be aware that things might change when you go back to your daily life. Don't wonder if the next few days feel a bit messy or chaotic. This is normal when we go through changes. Real change is an emotional process. Our body systems sort out things and reorganize themselves. Give yourself time, be patient with yourself, and be compassionate with yourself! Take this new awareness into your daily life and insert a bit of mindfulness every day. Before taking action, pause, breathe, relax, feel, and then go with the flow."

Every coin has two sides, and Anna started seeing the other side of the pain coin. One side is the dark shadow and distorsion. The other side is the golden shadow and light.Every story has two functions. I call the dark Shadow the parts of us that are more loaded with emotions of the lower and middle frequencies of the twenty-one tiers of emotions. I call the golden Shadow the parts of us that are loaded with the high frequencies of the tiers of emotions we don't allow to own.

What is the Shadow? Just as light illuminating an object also casts an area of darkness, said Carl Jung. The conscious brightness in how you see yourself creates a "Shadow"aspect of personality that goes unseen, like a blind spot. Attributes you think of as "bad"-feelings of anger, jealousy, hatred, fear, loneliness, and inferiority get relegated to your shadow and become unconscious.People who tend to focus on their negative characteristics and feelings with low energy and resonance, may hide some of their typically 'positive' feelings with high energy and resonance or qualities in their Shadow. The Shadow represents everything we refuse to acknowledge about ourselves that impacts the way we behave. Being blind to parts of ourselves means that there is often a difference between the person we think we are or the person we would like to see ourselves as and who we really are as we walk through the world. The Shadow is the aspect of ourselves that we have turned away from, ignored, and locked in the darkness. You can't see your Shadow, but you can feel it—and you can see your Shadow when you look into a mirror. The mirrors are the relationships we have with our spouses, partners, friends, colleagues, parents, and siblings. It is the part of ourselves we haven't owned and embraced yet. Very often, it is the part that becomes triggered in relationships and wants to be seen and integrated. We often repress our

Shadow aspects because they make us feel uncomfortable or bad about ourselves. But making these qualities unconscious gives them the power to create unintended impacts and problems in our lives and relationships when they influence us in ways we don't see. This unintended impact can also create pain in your body. These repressed aspects of your being might be the root of pain. Therefore Inner work is needed to reclaim the lost, fragmented parts of ourselves and integrate them. Developing our 'true' Self requires us to recognize, accept, and integrate all parts of ourselves, including our Shadow elements. My work can help you do that.

We all have Shadows. Nobody can do the Shadow and inner work for themselves! It's often found in emotional or physical pain. And very often, it's related to our family of origin.

Marianne Williamson said, "Our deepest fear is not that we are inadequate. Our deepest fear is that we are powerful beyond measure. It is our light, not our darkness that most frightens us."

Many people are afraid to shine and to own their brilliance to show this world. Integrating these missing elements of your shadow gives you more inner freedom and peace.

Do your shadow/inner work and own your own shit and brilliance. It's never too late to start. I'm naming the dark and light functions of our stories we are telling in our lives. These dark and light functions have nothing to do with the dark shadow and light/golden shadow. The stories we are telling have functions, and we can put them in dark and light functions.

The light function is revealing a need for healing and love, and it is empowering effort. It is taking responsibility for changing or creating our lives, trying new things, and learning new things. It is about possibilities and potential. It creates deeper intimate relationships, connections, and belonging.

The dark function is that we want to be rescued and are not taking responsibility for our own shit. We try to prove again and again that we are good enough and show how important we are. It can be addictive, and it creates separation. It has nothing to do with new awareness.

The dark side in us is called the negative ego. It creates separation. The shadow is the part that wants to be reclaimed. The dark side often stands in our way and controls us. It does not let us shine, and it pulls us down or back. The darkness isn't mean; it is only dark.

What's your biggest challenge in life? Can you turn it into a life you dream about? You can see the pain as a messenger who wants to be heard and seen to deliver different messages to us besides physical attention. It might be a stop sign to change the course of your life or the pain during the birth process. Giving birth to a new project by writing a book, building a business, changing careers, changing relationships, moving, or buying a house can cause pain. Imagine the pain of the physical birth process. It is not always a piece of cake. Pain might also be a simple hint to stop the cycle in your mind of negative, destructive thought patterns. *I'm not good enough. I'm not lovable. I'm not wanted. I'm not accepted. I'm not belonging.* It might be the stop sign of victimization.

Anna explored different options, and she figured out what the pain wanted to tell her. She faced her pain and engaged the pain. She understood the language of her pain, and she understood herself better. It was clear that it was a sign to change her life course and stop being a victim. It was a sign to break the cycle of her thought patterns: *I'm not good enough, and it is normal to be mistreated.* It was a sign to stop the belief that she deserves mistreatment instead of the sweetness of life. Anna needed to let go deeply. She needed to let go of her need to be in dysfunctional relationships and systems at work, in family relationships, in friendships, and in love relationships. She needed to become aware of that she has the birthright of aliveness, happiness, sweetness, success, joy, and peace. All of that came out in Anna's process, and it was all contained in her pain.

Everybody has a unique pain language that can be explored. It is everyone's decision and choice to start crossing the bridge from a cold, dark, painful place to the other side of warmth, light, and healing. Anna dreamed about getting rid of the pain and feeling much better. She was ready for the journey across the bridge. Everyone can go when the time is right.

Anna decided to fight for her birthright and fight for love. That fight emerged from her soul instead of saying "I must, I should, I have to."

She was longing for more in life, and she broke free from repression, suppression, and victimization. It was beautiful to see her vulnerable inner warrior for love coming out.

I love my work with my clients. One of my passions is guiding them on the hero journey to the other side of the bridge. Processing our feelings and thoughts is not something we learn in school or at home. We have to learn it on our own.

CHAPTER

7

THE PAIN LIVES IN THE CHAKRAS

"WHAT IS A chakra?" Anna asked.

I was telling Anna about energy lives in our chakra systems, but she didn't know what I meant. "It takes time to experience the energy we don't see. It is the subtlest energy that is unseen, untouchable, and invisible. You cannot smell it, hear it neither feel it. You only can sense it in terms of an inner, intuitive knowing.

Chakra means wheel, and it is the center of activity in us. It receives, conforms, and expresses life force energy. These are centers in the subtle body where emotions and thoughts come together and affect the next level, the physical body. This plays a role in how we interact with others and the outside world.

The chakra system is the relationship between the physical body and psychological body, our psyche and soma (body). Here is an example how chakras work. Let's say we experience emotional fear. Fear is related to our first chakra at the base of the spine. We have seven main chakras in our bodies.

Fear can show up in our bodies in different ways: shortness of breath, butterflies in our stomachs, shaky voices, or sweaty hands. This lack of confidence might lead us to be treated in a way that is harmful and perpetuates the fear. The fear could have its roots in an unresolved and unhealed childhood experience that still influences our behaviors and how people react to us and treat us. Anna was mistreated by her husband, her boss, and her father. Her fear was related to unresolved and unhealed wounds. That energy was working subconsciously, and she was sending it out into the world and attracting people who hooked her in relationships that caused harm and destruction rather than love and compassion.

Working with the chakras means healing ourselves. Old wounds are locked in the cells of our tissues and minds. For Anna, it was back pain and neck pain.

The seven chakras are big centers with wheels. They build one main column along the spine, and they are connected by energy tracts that are like superhighways in our bodies. The energy travels from one center to the next one. These vital centers are like gas stations in our bodies that provide energy, gas, and vital force of consciousness. They lift or slow our energy. This unseen energy can be felt in exercises that make us aware of the sensations in our bodies. On a physical level, our chakras communicate with our nervous systems and hormone systems. The seven chakras are associated with seven basic levels of consciousness.

Each chakra also holds a shadow. Chakras send energy from inside out and receive energy from outside in. They organize life energy. It is common to become trapped in any patterns in our lives, and as a consequence, we may stay stuck in them. We can learn to direct or redirect the patterns and break the cycle to get them unstuck.

Anna was stuck in two of her chakras. She was caught up in the cycle of her marriage and her thought patterns. Other cycles where we can be caught up can be relationships, jobs, habits, or ways of thinking. Being trapped in a pattern means being stuck in a chakra. Being stuck can appear as an overemphasis or underdevelopment of a chakra. And chakras can show in physical reactions. For instance, Anna was stuck in her fifth chakra, and that showed up in tightness and pain in her neck. That chakra is also associated with communication. Anna stopped communicating and suppressed her feelings in her marriage before she came out and broke the silence.

The intention is to clean these chakras so the life energy can flow freely through them and they can open and close flexibly in response to situations.

For many of my clients, the work with the chakra system is new. It was also new to Anna, and she was very surprised to experience the connection between the energy, the stickiness in her life, her symptoms, her pain, and the life issues that were sitting in her chakras and causing her pain. She was stuck in her third and fifth chakra.

A short overview of the seven chakras and their associated elements in nature and the shadow side may explain the quality of the chakra and Anna's experience.

Chakra One

- Location: base of the spine
- Association: survival
- Element: earth
- Shadow: fear
- Malfunction: obesity, anorexia, sciatica, constipation
- Reflection Questions: Do you consider yourself well grounded? How often do you prepare your own food? How is your relationship to money and work?
- Affirmations: I love my body and trust its wisdom. I choose to take responsibility for looking after myself in all ways.

Chakra 2

- Location: lower abdomen
- Association: emotions and sexuality
- Element: water
- Shadow: guilt
- Malfunction: sexual problems, urinary trouble
- Reflection questions: How would you rate your sex life? How would you rate your ability to feel and express your emotions? How much time do you create for simple pleasure in life? How would you rate your emotional and physical flexibility?
- Affirmations: I deserve the pleasure in my life. I enjoy my body and feel good about my sexuality.

Chakra 3

- Location: solar plexus
- Association: personal power, self-esteem
- Element: fire
- Shadow: shame
- Malfunction: digestive system, liver, gall bladder, digestive trouble, chronic fatigue, hypertension
- Reflection questions: How would you rate your digestion? How would you see yourself in being reliable? How confident are you?
- Affirmations: I can do whatever I want to do. I value who I am. The fire within me burns through all the blocks and fears.

Chakra 4

- Location: over the sternum (the heart center)
- Association: love
- Element: air
- Shadow: grief, resentment
- Malfunction: lungs, heart, circulatory system, arms, hands, asthma, coronary disease, lung disease
- Reflection questions: What's your relationship in loving yourself? Do you love yourself? What's your capacity in forgiving past hurts from others? Can you be true to your feelings? Can you love someone as they are without expecting them to change for you? What's your relationship with compassion? Can you feel compassion for those with faults and troubles?
- Affirmations: I open my heart and accept others as who they are. I release my pain and forgive the past. I'm free to love. I'm worthy of love.

Chakra 5

- Location: throat
- Association: communication and creativity
- Element: sound
- Shadow: lies

- Malfunction: throat, ears, mouth, shoulders, neck, sore throat, neck and shoulder pain, thyroid troubles
- Reflection questions: What is your relationship to your creative side? How often do you speak up for yourself and speak your truth? What kind of listener are you?
- Affirmations: Creativity is my birthright. My voice matters. I speak from my heart. I speak up for myself.

Chakra 6

- Location: center of the forehead between the eyes (third eye)
- Association: intuition and imagination
- Element: light
- Shadow: illusion
- Malfunction: Vision problems, headaches, nightmares
- Reflection questions: What is your dream? How would you rate your ability to visualize? Can you see the bigger picture of your life? Do you have a vision for your life?
- Affirmations: I am open to my wisdom within. I am open to my intuition. I forgive myself for my own limitations.

Chakra 7

- Location: top of the head
- Association: knowledge, wisdom, understanding, and consciousness
- Element: thought
- Shadow: attachment
- Malfunction: depression, confusion
- Reflection questions: What's your relationship with meditation? Do you meditate? What's your openness to other ways of being or thinking? How easy is it for you to work through attachments and release them? What's your purpose and meaning in life?
- Affirmations: I'm guided by higher power and inner wisdom. I am love, truth, freedom, and beauty. I am love. I am joy. I am freedom. Gratitude awakens the good to unfold in my life.

The chakras can be open, closed, or between. That is common when it is working free. It can also stuck in a closed way or an open way. Anna was stuck primarily in her third chakra. A closed chakra is a chronic avoidance of energies and running on low energy, and an excessively open chakra is a chronic fixation and running on high energy.

The intention is to balance the energy in the chakras between high and low and clean the energy whenever we are in the way of low energy such as depression or high energy such as restlessness and anxiety. The lower chakras contain information about survival, sexuality, and action. The higher chakras bring us more states of consciousness and the belief system about spirituality, meaning, and living a purposeful life.

Anna's pain situation sucked energy and resulted in low energy and partly depressive moods. Her third chakra—the seat of power, willpower and self-esteem—was blocked. She felt powerless. Many of my clients who were blocked in their third chakras felt powerless, helpless, frustrated, and angry. These are all related feelings, and energy held back in this chakra causes body pain and polarities in low energy or high energy, showing up in depression or anxiety.

If Anna was not determined to work on herself and her issues, it would have cost her mental health and showed up in long-term depression or anxiety. Her feelings of being victimized, trapped, powerless, helpless, and frustrated were all sitting in the third chakra. It is the element of fire. The fire helps us digest and burns blockades away, but her fire was not burning because the center was blocked. She was stuck in the center. People were stepping over her boundaries. She was not setting healthy boundaries. Her husband was stepping over Anna's boundaries. He stepped on Anna's feet and was staying there. It was painful, but he held the power of removing his foot. The pain was Anna's, and she had the responsibility to start to set boundaries and tell her husband to stop stepping on her feet. The learning of saying no lies in the willpower and self-esteem of this chakra.

Many of my clients tend to over-give and miss out to take care of themselves and say no and set boundaries. Anna learned to develop a sense of self. She identified her needs and desires, and she started to communicate them. She stepped into her willpower and into her fire energy. She developed a great connection to her body. She listened and sensed herself and felt if her body showed a green light, a yellow light, or a red light. She used her body as the core instrument of her truth. Whenever she was not able to sense her body, she paused, relaxed, and took a few breaths. She was noticing her breathing. It is the connection and bridge between the physical body and mental/emotional body, and it helped her ground herself and feel herself again whenever she was disconnected.

"I'm noticing a big change in my body. My pain is less, and I feel much better. The nights are getting better, my sleep is deeper, and I can get up in the morning without pain. I feel the biggest challenge and opportunity in my present life is to say no to things I don't want, set my boundaries, and change my old patterns. I notice how good it feels and how my body reacts, and it shows I'm on the right track. At the same time, I can see how people, especially my husband, react to my new behavior. It influences me, and I know I need to stay committed to myself. My husband, my children, my friends, and my colleagues are not used to my new behavior."

"Of course," I said. "Their reactions are normal."

I notice the same reaction with many of my clients. When they change, their environment changes too. For some, it is convenient, and for others, it is not.

"You do not have to control your husband's reaction to your process of self-care," I said. "That is not your responsibility. People will react when you change or when you do things differently. It affects them in some way. Let them have their feelings, let them have their reactions, and continue on your course."

Anna continued to her self-mastery, and she nurtured herself.

I showed her how to say no gracefully, which is useful for marriages, friends, children, families, and careers.

CHAPTER

8

⸻———————————————●

EIGHT KEYS TO
MASTERING
YOURSELF

*If we do not observe ourselves, we cannot
ever hope to be our own master.*
—Don Richard Riso

ANNA WAS 100 percent committed to her path of healing and change, and her pain had decreased, she felt relaxed, and her sleep was restful. Although it required a lot of inner work and the whole issue with her marriage came on the surface, she knew she would not run away from it. The cost would be too high for her. Although she did not know the outcome of her marriage, she was accountable to herself to work on her issues and to clean up her inner house. That was a big recognition, and I was happy she noticed it.

I know how difficult it can be if you don't know what will happen and you need to trust the process and surrender into it. I know it from my own experience and with many of my clients. Anna's starting point was the same, and she experienced some key steps that helped her release the physical pain and underlying emotional pain.

She said, "I was so covered and blocked in my pain that I could not see and feel what I had created in my life when I came here the first time. I had no clue what would happen, and to be honest, I was also afraid. There were times I wanted to run away, but the urgency, pain, and suffering were so high that I kept going. By the time I recognized what was going on in my life, my awareness had grown. The healing work of my inner child and the wounds and shadow work were key elements in the process of seeing my unique story in life. It was a very emotional process. I learned to feel myself and get out of numbness and not feeling. I learned to listen to my body and the voice of my pain. I'm still learning to identify my voices and master my destructive mind talk. I'm still exploring myself, the peace of self-acceptance—and what it means to me—and forgiveness. My marriage has changed. It still has ups and downs, but overall, I feel much better. I feel like I'm back to myself—to my new self. I feel I'm different in the same situation. I can feel a shift in my inner world, and the situations with my husband and work might be less painful."

That was a big step in growing and developing herself for the sake of letting go of pain!

Here are the eight steps Anna took in her process of mastering herself:

STEP 1

Key 1: Taking Responsibility

A four-step model based on Lucid Living (www.lucidliving.net; www.greatstorycoaching.com):

- Recognize: Develop awareness of how you create the circumstances in your life and accept life as it is. Life is our curriculum.
- Acknowledge: Take responsibility and ownership of what you are creating, experience the range of emotions that are related to these circumstances, and feel the emotions and the impact of your decisions and choices on you and others. Experience the secret of your emotions.
- Forgive: Develop and experience understanding and forgiveness and feel it in your body.
- Change: Experience the change you wish to create and make a commitment to manifest the change.

Key 2: Healthy Boundaries as a Nurturing Parent

Learn to accept what was in the past and set healthy boundaries for the future. Say no to things you don't want and need, and that is nonnegotiable. Say yes to things you want and are passionate about. Determine where you can negotiate and compromise. Learn to set boundaries with clarity and grace. Articulate and do not be afraid to name what's going on. The more you come from your heart, the easier it is. Become aware of who you want to be and who you are not. Say no to things that are not you. Say yes because this is who you are and want to be. Sometimes it is enough to develop the security to be able to say no. Seek people who have healthy boundaries and who are modeling healthy boundaries. Practicing compassion with yourself is part of setting boundaries.

Key 3: Identify Your Valuable Voices

Think of yourself as the CEO or king or queen in your house or castle, and there are all these different voices sitting at the table for a meeting in your house. These are all your team members, and all of them are the voices of your mind. Who is sitting at the table? Which voice is talking to you? Is it the critic parent, the saboteur, the controller, the observer, the appreciator, the inner child, the loving, compassionate nurturing parent, the victim, the striver, or the conscious creator? Who are they?

And remember that you are in charge. The king/queen/CEO makes the final decisions.

HOW TO IDENTIFY YOUR INNER VOICES

The different voices are related to feelings and body sensations. Start to determine if your body feels open, relaxed, and free. Is breathing easy? If your muscles feel constricted or under tension, your breath isn't free.

- Self-sabotaging/gremlin voices: critic parent or controller who creates tension, constriction, and shortness of breath, withholding breath, stop breathing.
- Observer: neutral, nonjudgmental, and creates openness and free breath in your body.
- Appreciator: filled with gratitude and acknowledgment and creates openness, relaxation, and free breath in your body.
- Criticized Inner child: creates constriction and openness in your body. A vulnerable child or a magic or playful child will determine what feelings are running through your body. For instance, fear and excitement create different reactions in your body.
- Nurturing inner parent: compassionate and understanding and create relaxation, openness, and free breathing in your body.
- Victim: creates openness or restriction in your body, depending on the dark or light function of your victim story.
- Striver: creates openness or restriction in your body, depending on the dark or light function of your striver story.
- Conscious creator: creates openness in your body and free breathing.

After you've practiced distinguishing the body sensations and feelings, you can move over to step 2 to identify your inner voices:

STEP 2

- Whenever you feel constriction or resistance in your body, check what messages, words, sentences you are receiving.
- Whenever you feel openness in your heart or body, check what messages, sentences, and words are coming up and crossing your mind.
- Start to explore and figure out who is talking to you. Is it your victim voice, striver voice, saboteur/critical/controlling parent, inner child, observer, or appreciator? Are all of them talking at the same time? Who's talking loudest in this moment? Who is taking the lead and driving the bus?

- Let them communicate with each other and create an inner team meeting.
- The saboteur, critical/controlling parent says, "You are not good enough."
- The appreciator says, "You did a great job."
- The nurturing parent says, "I love you. I hear you. I see you."
- The observer says, "I notice you're angry, sad, or joyful."
- The vulnerable, wounded inner child screams, "I'm hurting. I feel lonely. I'm scared, I don't belong."
- The conscious creator adult says, "I'm hurting."
- The victim voice (dark function) says, "Why is this always happening to me?"
- The striver says, "I need to finish this and that before I can relax."

Some voices are so quiet that you barely hear them. You need to develop consciousness and mindfulness to recognize them and invite them to speak their truth loudly. It makes sense to learn to identify the voices with an experienced coach since the nuances between some voices are so fine that it is hard to learn on your own. Invest at least once on a coach—there's nothing to lose. Once you're trained and familiar with them, it gets easy to recognize. It is a lot of fun, it is fulfilling, and it makes you feel more alive!

Key 4: Heal Your Core Wounds and Your Inner Child

We all have a little child within us. It is an essential part of our being. It can be playful, vulnerable, or magical. The more we understand that inner child, the more we understand who we are and why we are here. This inner child is the part and energy in all of us that remembers why we are here. Through our inner child, you will know your purpose in life.

Our childhood experiences affect our thoughts, belief systems, and emotions. It is crucial to healing unresolved wounds. Otherwise, it will continue to act out and contaminate our adult lives. When our feelings are suppressed or repressed, especially anger or pain, we grow up with an angry, hurt child inside us. We may react to others instead of responding.

The wounded inner child is a major cause of problems in our individual lives and in the world. We all have small or big wounds in us. Some of them are unresolved, nag at us, and cause pain. People may trigger them if they are not healed. As long as they are not healed, they prevent us from creating deep, loving, intimate connections and relationships. They mask the core Self, the truest Self, and the soul. They keep us holding on to what happened in the past and attach us to old patterns. They prevent us away from moving forward and living in the present. Being trapped with our thoughts from the past may cause depression, and being too much in our thoughts about the future may cause fear and anxiety. Living in the here and now lets us feel connected and expansive, and it can create different levels of intimate connections when our wounds are healed.

The inner child is the part of you that holds your memories, your soul, your deepest thoughts, and your feelings. Getting to know your inner child helps you understand you better. It helps you accept and love yourself. Understanding ourselves is essential to a peaceful, joyous, and pain-free life.

Key 5: Facing Your Shadow

Do Your Shadow/Inner work and own your own shit and brilliance. It's never too late to start with it. The Shadow is the aspect of ourselves and our souls that we have turned away from, ignored, and locked into the darkness. It is the part of ourselves we haven't owned and embraced yet.

We all have Shadow. Nobody can do the shadow and inner work alone! We have a dark Shadow or a golden Shadow. Some people have locked in their feelings of fear, shame, and anger, and some have locked in their feelings of brilliance, joy, and success. It's often noticed in emotional or physical pain, and it's often related to our family of origin.

Most of the time, fear is a basic human Shadow. Fear of death, loss, rejection, conflict, confrontation, or failure—and even fear of success—are always running unconsciously in the background.

Once you have faced and integrated these missing elements of your Shadow, it gives you more inner freedom and peace and healing from pain.

Key 6: Trust the process!

Key 7: As soon as you physically shift your emotional state, your psyche will follow!

Key 8: Read The Four Agreements *by Don Miguel Ruiz and* Healing Your Aloneness *by Erika J. Chopich and Margaret Paul.*

We can change from both sides as well as from inside out and outside in. The physical body has an impact on the psyche, and the psyche influences the physical body.

Linda was a single woman in her thirties, and she was a social worker in a hospital. She was highly sensitive, and she had chronic back pain, neck pain, and pain in her knees. The issues sitting in her tissues were her situation as a single woman with a baby wish, feeling unsatisfied in her job, conflicts with her boss, and the loss of her mom. There were times she came with low energy and pain in her neck or lower back. After she started working on these issues, all the pain became secondary.

She went through all the steps above, and I started to dream and explore visions with her. In one session, Linda started dreaming. Her dream was working for a season on a cottage in the mountains and leaving her job and the conflicts at work. She was passionate about nature and the mountains. A year later, her dream came true. She was so brave to quit her job, follow her dream, and work the summer season at the cottage on the mountain. She said, "I will come back and see what happens regarding a new job."

What trust she had in herself and life! She decided to change the course of her life. I was in awe of her trust and courage. It was amazing to witness. It was not necessary to quit her job because she negotiated getting the time off for the summer and could go back to her job and look for a new job from there. It was amazing. Her dream was sitting in the pain of her neck, back, and knee.

And when she came back from the cottage, she said, "I'm fine. In fact, I'm even better than I've been in a long time. I go to work without being particularly touched or stressed out. I decided not to do the next certification program. Instead, I'm taking time for myself to live and enjoy life. I have begun to separate the desire for a partnership from my desire to have children. The considerations are still very much in the beginning, but in principle, I have the idea that this is not necessarily coherent. I could do it alone, which creates infinite serenity and freedom. I nurture my body and listen to my soul. I do more yoga, which helps me feel like me, and I'm mindful of food and pay attention to eat well. My heart is full of gratitude. A thousand thanks for guiding me on my inner journey in the past few years. Through your companionship, I have been able to learn very impressively and sustainably how much wisdom is in the body, how much the body speaks, nonverbally and how important just listening is."

I love how Linda developed a deep compassion for herself. I love my work. I love serving my clients and guiding them on their hero journeys!

We do not always allow ourselves to work through pain. More often than not, we think pain is a signal that we must stop, rather than find its source. Our souls aspire toward growth, that is, toward remembering all that we have forgotten due to our trip to this place, the earth. In this context, a body in pain is a soul in longing.
—Malidoma Patrice Somé

CHAPTER
9

NOURISH YOURSELF

"WHAT CAN I do in my daily life?" Anna asked. "I'm here today and am feeling much, much better. I'm more relaxed and feel no pain anymore. I don't want to be back into this horrible cycle."

I responded, "I love that you are taking care of yourself, Anna, and that your well-being has become so important for you. You did a great job with your process and who you have become!"

Here are a few pieces of advice about how you can continue to nurture yourself. Nurturing yourself and becoming your own nurturing parent is the key. A lot of compassion is required on a daily basis.

You have changed yourself from inside out, and this change needs to be applied to your daily life. Your daily style of living needs to be adapted and changed too. That means that you need to change from outside in too.

How can you do this?

Here are six keys to integrate easily on a daily basis and nourish yourself:

MINDFULNESS KEY 1

Begin your day mindfully. Take at least five minutes in the morning for yourself with a cup of coffee or tea or in meditation. Use this five minutes to greet the new day intentionally and set your intention for the day. Decide how you want to be and feel that day. Setting intentions is different from setting goals and has different effects.

MINDFULNESS KEY 2

Pause, relax, breathe, and feel. Insert a moment of mindfulness in your day before any action. Check in at least three times a day and wonder if you are still connected with your breath. Ground yourself, regulate yourself and center yourself daily. Just observe and sense your cycle of inhalation and exhalation. There's nothing more to do. Isn't that simple, and it is free! You don't need to pay anything besides paying attention to yourself and giving yourself a few seconds or minutes a day. And you can integrate it wherever you are: in a meeting, driving, or standing in line at the grocery store.

The effect is strong if you're doing it on a regular basis and integrate it into your life. Make a routine out of it, such as when you're brushing your teeth every day. The breathing connects us, it connects our bodies and minds, and it influences our nervous systems, hormone systems, and digestive systems. It reduces the release of stress hormones and pain hormones.

When we are in states of change, we often forget to breathe or hold our breath. This can happen even when changing positions. Try it out by observing yourself in these moments. For instance, when you get up from a stool and walk into the kitchen, are you still breathing? Are you aware of your breathing? Try a different way of getting up. We're often more focused on things outside of ourselves than on what is inside of us.

The breath is the bridge between the physical body and the subtle body. It connects our bodies, minds, and souls. Breathing gives us life!

MINDFULNESS KEY 3

Complete your day mindfully. Before you go to bed and close your eyes, take a few moments to answer these questions:

- What was fun today?
- What went well today? Where did I succeed? And success can be everything—even little things!
- What am I grateful for?

You can share these questions and answers with your spouse or partner. It is fun and creates a different space of intimacy. If you are sharing it with a partner or spouse, you may also ask, "What did I appreciate about you today?"

MINDFULNESS KEY 4

Stay grounded. You can practice a grounding exercise every morning, and it is highly supportive to do it before an important meeting, an important conversation with your boss, or for conflict resolution in a relationship or at work.

MINDFULNESS KEY 5

Practice mindful eating. With Anna, we also checked in with her nutrition patterns. Stress and pain are the enemies in our bodies, and they like to eat up some important vitamins and affect our metabolic cycles. Vitamin B is one example that is very often affected.

When we are in change and processing or digesting a lot of emotions, mental patterns, or behaviors, we need a nutritional balance and boost. Anna was not processing her issues and then going home and drinking multiple glasses of wine or eating bunches of chocolate. That is counterproductive, and I experienced it with some of my other clients. It has to do with setting healthy boundaries regarding food and taking care of yourself.

MINDFULNESS KEY 6

Cleansings. I advise a ten-day Ayurvedic cleansing once or twice a year! Ayurveda is the extraordinary mind-body medicine of India. Its great yogic spiritual traditions bring wholeness to all levels of our existence. It is one of the oldest and most complete systems of natural healing worldwide, and it contains great wisdom for all human beings

Cleansing on a regular basis is part of taking care of your physical body, your emotional body, and your mental body. It is giving a gift to yourself. Detoxification is just as necessary for the body as for the mind. To begin detoxification, we must first stop taking toxins into ourselves. Fasting from food helps detoxify the body, and fasting from impressions detoxifies your mind. The food we eat affects our bodies, but it also affects our entire state of mind. The quality of our food becomes the quality of our consciousness. Unless we change our eating behaviors, we are unlikely to be able to change our consciousness. If we want to get rid of pain, reduce inflammation, raise our consciousness, and calm our emotions, we cannot ignore the food we eat.

Cleansings are great breaks to stop cycles and raise awareness regarding food and get rid of pain. You can integrate this ten-day ayurvedic cleansing program into your busy life, and you can do it from home. My busy clients can integrate it into their busy lives.

I've experimented with different cleansing and fast programs. This is a great in-between solution if you don't have time to take a break for four to six weeks to do a long cleansing program. It is a soft approach to fasting. The impact of a soft cleansing is to balance and clean your digestive fire—the channels of your metabolic system—and strengthen your organs and tissue. It supports letting go of toxic elements in your tissues, activates your circulation, releases water, and enhances the metabolic functions of your body. Consequently, your immunity and self-healing forces increase. It grounds you and gives you energy, strength, and vitality.

From the Ayurvedic perspective, it is not recommended to do a total fast with only water for more than one and a half days. There are only a few exceptions where it makes sense to fast only with water. Otherwise, it will change your metabolism so that your digestive fire will slow down completely—and it will increase your energy in a direction that is less grounded.

The ten days are divided into four phases, and all of the phases have an effect of cleansing. It is all based on mung beans, which have a high efficiency of detoxification. There's one day with only drinking water included.

It is a great experience and great time to cleanse your body on all levels. The cleansings always affect your emotional and mental body. It is a time to let go of toxic elements in your physical body and toxic thought patterns and beliefs. It is especially highly recommended after intense coaching processes or retreats.

I recommend doing it at least once a year and twice if possible. The best time for cleansing is when the seasons are changing. The transition from winter to spring or from late summer to fall are best for me. It helps you let go of things from the past season and get you ready for the next season. It encourages your body to let go of pain for good.

At the end of this book, you will find a link to the ten-day Ayurvedic cleansing program. Please reach out and send me an email if you have any questions!

These are the main keys I recommend integrating on a daily basis. Try to process it, digest it in your body and brain, and understand it intellectually. Go out into nature as often as possible. Nature has a very healing effect on us.

Sign up for a body movement practice that slows your body and encourages you to go deeper into your inner world and connect with your emotional/mental body, the subtle body. Yoga and meditation both slow your body, and yoga is the only approach I know that has an impact on all five layers. As a yoga and meditation instructor, I know the positive effects on pain, stress, emotions, depression, and anxiety. I highly recommend practicing them at least once a week. It is good to do something for your body that has an effect on your cardio system; try running, swimming, walking, or hiking.

Anna said, "I need to do something with my body. I need to feel my body. I can't do only processing my stuff in coaching and my brain."

I fully agreed. We need to integrate what we are processing into our bodies. She signed up for yoga and meditation, and it gave her a great boost and moved her forward in the process of letting go of the pain.

Here is a summary of daily/weekly nourishments:

- mindful start of a new day
- mindful completion of a day
- mindful eating
- mindful breathing breaks
- mindful grounding

- going out into nature
- yoga to connect with the five layers of your body
- meditation to calm your mind and slow down
- swimming, running, walking, or hiking for cardio activation
- optional: journaling (see the benefits of journaling in chapter 5 p.41)

The challenge for Anna was scheduling all these breaks for herself and making it happen despite her busy daily life with children, job, and husband. She was aware of what the cost would be if she did not radically change her lifestyle. And she did it! She showed commitment, accountability, respect, and self-discipline. She has fallen in love with herself and developed a major skill—*compassion*—which is the bridge and weapon of pain. Love and compassion are the new pill of the twenty-first century. They kill the pain. Love is the painkiller.

And here are a few things you can try to integrate into your daily life. These optional things have a powerful impact on healing! Have you ever done journaling?

Journaling is a tool I offered Anna as homework, and she loved it. It helped her connect with her creative side and cultivate inner dialogues with herself. At the beginning of her journey, she did it every day. She really liked it because it was a way to let her unexpressed emotions out by writing them down. It opened a door for her, and she unlocked her emotions. She wrote them down in a beautiful book she chose for herself as another act of self-love.

Anna said, "It is a special time when I'm sitting there with a cup of tea, a candle in front of me, and I'm journaling in my beautiful book. It is a date with myself, and I enjoy the time of conscious stream."

You can do journaling in different ways and with different intentions. You can journal about a question or do a conscious stream. There are many options. I encourage you to experience it and practice it for at least four weeks.

Have you ever worked with affirmations, statements, or the Enneagram? This is a powerful tool that supported Anna's process and self-development.

Anna said, "I'm using my chakra affirmation every morning as an intentional start. It reminds me of my strength and power, and at the same time, it sets down my old thoughts and belief patterns that were sucking my energy and causing pain and suffering. It boosts my energy and connects me to myself."

While I was training with Lucid Living, we created statements that were very powerful affirmations. I create them with my clients and find their unique words.

Don Richard Riso developed the Enneagram and Enneagram transformations. Knowing your Enneagram type helps you become a more conscious leader and observer. The combination of affirmations and statements can be very impactful on your life. It is created out of your own words and writing down a certain thought pattern or belief. You will show up with a stronger commitment in your daily life, and you will feel freer.

Have you ever dared to daydream again? In childhood, we are so used to dreaming, but in adulthood, we lost dreaming. Dreaming is beautiful. In a dreaming session, Anna went into her dream body. She was totally lost in her body, and she connected with her pain and transformed it by getting out essential messages about herself. Dreaming transported her to another mood, and that energy helped her escape the pain. Dreaming can feed your new story and your new identity. What are you dreaming about?

A NOTE FOR HIGHLY SENSITIVE PEOPLE

In one of the last chapters, I talked specifically about highly sensitive people and pain. In this chapter, I also offered a self-nourishment plan. For those who already know or assume that they are highly sensitive, I recommend following the plan in the HSP chapter and adding things from the advice above. I hope you find a way to nourish yourself and take great care of yourself on a daily basis! If you need help getting started, and want to learn more about ways to relieve stress and pain, contact me to schedule a consultation – the first step to a healthier you. Email at ab@ annabelle-breuer.com

CHAPTER
10

THE POWER
OF RITUALS

*A ritual is an enactment of a myth. And, by participating in the
ritual, you are paricipating in the myth. And since myth is a
projection of the depth wisdom of the psyche, by participating in
a ritual, participating in the myth, you are being, as it were, put
in accord with that wisdom, which is the wisdom that is inherent
within you anyhow. Your consciousness is being, reminded of the
wisdom of your own life. I think ritual is terribly important.*
—Joseph Campbell

MY HUSBAND AND I did a beautiful ritual before our marriage. We found a quiet spot on a lake and sat on stones. We were the only ones there, and we shared what we let go and didn't want to take into our marriage and what we invited and would bring into our marriage. It was very powerful to witness my husband sharing his intimate thoughts and emotions, and it was vulnerable for me to open my heart and share my thoughts and feelings.

Rituals are powerful tools that support us to invite and manifest new raw materials, thoughts, dreams, and visions and let go of old material. Rituals sharpen our consciousness regarding a certain theme, and they help us heal and intentionally integrate what's happening around us. There are different rituals for different events. For instance, it is impactful in times of healing from pain, career or relationship transitions, or moving to a new city or country. It is wonderful to use rituals to strengthen the bonding in a love relationship or for important projects. It can be used to confirm an ending of a relationship or a certain time of life. There are rituals to transform burdensome emotions and pain that stick with us and determine or control us. There are many opportunities to experience the magic and power from a ritual.

Most of my clients like the idea and practice of rituals. I used rituals after my divorce and before I moved from Germany to the United States.

Anna was new to the lesson of rituals and was very curious about them. She asked, "What does it have to do with getting rid of the pain?"

"Rituals support us in the healing process and in feeling much better and in letting go of pain," I responded. "It helps us create a new present. The future creates the present—not the past. For that reason, it makes sense to let go of old things and invite the new things and new raw materials to manifest in the new present."

I did a letting go ritual with Anna. She let go of things that were no longer serving her. If we let go of a phase in our lives or a job or a partner, we say goodbye to positive experiences and negative experiences. All of it is passed from the moment we let go. Anna was clear that she wanted to let go of her old pattern of trying to please everybody and striving through life until she was exhausted or in pain again. We did the ritual of letting go to mark an important ending and a new beginning in her life. At the same time, we invited her new raw material to practice setting healthy boundaries.

What did the ritual look like? First, she created a list of yeses and nos in her life to become clearly aware of what she wants to let go of and what she wants to invite into her life. Anna chose a wide pink band and made knots in the ribbon for all she experienced in that phase of her life. Be sure that the band is long enough. She tied it to an end in her home, and every day, she took a few minutes and thought about what she wanted to let go of. She cut a piece that was as big as she felt appropriate to let go. Some days, she could cut more off because she felt really angry and wanted to leave it all behind her, and on other days, it was only possible to cut a little piece off since she held onto old things and was still attached to them.

I said, "Anytime you cut a piece off, be aware of what you are feeling and sensing in your body. Be compassionate with yourself and trust the process that the day will come when you have let go completely."

Anna worked on the list of her yeses and nos in our sessions. She let go of the nos during her daily ritual at home, and we worked on the yeses for the new raw materials in her new phase of life. The yes list was integrated into another ritual. It was a powerful celebration ritual and a ritual of new beginnings. You can repeat a ritual until a shift of the issue, theme, or pattern is felt in your life. It takes time to get used to it and develop the consciousness around it. It also takes openness and beliefs in the practice of rituals and magic. You can invite the magical and playful side of your inner child.

Anna's homework kept her moving forward on her journey.

I said, "Create a passion list and gratitude list with at least twenty things you are passionate about and twenty-one things you are grateful for in life."

With her passion list, we started to create a passion statement to feed her new story, her new identity, and her new phase of life. The gratitude list helped her shift perspectives, and she started to see things in her life through a different lens. She could see much more beauty in her life. I suggested creating a gratitude jar to use at home with her family. Whenever they are up for it, they pick a small piece of paper and write done what they are grateful for. It can be shared before they put it into the jar. It is a fun and bonding experience to share it with somebody, and it cultivates intimacy in any relationship.

Gratitude is one of the most healing and powerful vibrations. It contains elements of feeling thankful, joyful, happy, creative, vulnerable, and loving. The intention of a gratitude ritual is to bring awareness to the vibrancy of the elements of gratitude and cultivate those feelings frequently.

Anna's life was not full of gratitude, and she was not open to seeing it until she went through her process. Most of her days were gray, and she was convinced that things and people outside of herself held the key to happiness and freedom from pain. When Anna tried to control the situation, she was trapped. People and things can't stop our pain or heal us. Anna became aware of that she needed to take responsibility to change her situation. In the end, her pain transported her to a state of gratitude and compassion. She learned that one simple thing like being open to seeing what she was thankful for could move her through a stressful time. It helped her stop trying to control outcomes. It helped her be more relaxed and serene and to surrender into daily situations. It helped her turn her pain into joy and freedom. We don't have sunny days every day. Gray days in between are normal, and they belonging to us. If Anna's pain is coming back on a gray day, she knows to stop and listen to her body.

Those are the days when old feelings and patterns come rushing back and want to take over. We are not the same every day, and we are not always in the same mood of high energy and vibration. However, it makes a difference how and who we are on a gray day. On gray days, Anna knows the sun is still shining behind the clouds. Even in shady times, the sun is still there. Even when it is cloudy and gray, she can see the beauty inside and outside of herself. And when her pain is coming back on a gray day, she knows she needs to stop, slow down, and listen to her body and the message of her pain. She needs to take time to take care of herself, and she needs to be aware of her thoughts.

Robert A. Emmons, PhD, the world's leading scientific expert on gratitude said, "Gratitude has the power to heal, energize, and change lives."

CHAPTER
11

THE BIG OBSTACLES

*Without leaps of imagination or dreaming, we lose the excitement
of possibilities. Dreaming, after all, is a form of planning.*
—Gloria Steinem

ON GRAY DAYS, old feelings, old patterns, and pain want to take over our lives. When you started reading this book, the process started in you. Those days are normal, and obstacles are coming your way. These obstacles might challenge you. They might challenge you to ask for help in processing it. They might challenge you to see if you are still committed to yourself and your well-being and living a healthy life. In this chapter, I want to prepare you for those days.

What is needed? From my point of view, coaching is needed! I've seen how effective coaching is for releasing pain. I have witnessed it in hundreds of my clients' lives, and I've guided and helped them through painful times and phases. At least once in your life, invest in a few coaching sessions to set the foundation and groundwork. The investment is worth it, and you are working on self-care and self-love. From time to time, I still have a coach to clean up my own things, check if I'm still on the path of my heart and soul, and see if I'm purposefully following my calling. It is really supportive!

Set your healthy boundaries and use the four steps of responsibility to identify and manage your voices. The universe and outside situations will always challenge us and see if we are ready for the next lesson in our lives. This is how I see life. Life is our curriculum, and life is about challenges.

In these situations, the pain can come back or get worse. It can wake us up to more consciousness.

Nadine was forty years old, and she lived in California with her husband and two children. Right after her first child was born, she came to me with bad lower back pain. It was not only the physical pain of giving birth. This pain contained feelings of not being enough at work, conflicts with her boss, not feeling seen and heard at work, and not feeling acknowledged. The old issue of the divorce of her parents resurfaced. She compensated for the emotional pain by eating, and that had an impact on her body and lower back pain.

Whenever she felt emotionally stressed out, she started eating chocolate and more sugar, and her portions became bigger. During the coaching process, she learned to notice what was happening and to become aware of and acknowledge her feelings. She was able to take responsibility for her actions and consciously make decisions and choices. Whenever she was in emotional turmoil, she paused, took a few breaths, and felt into herself, her body, and the situation. She relaxed before she took action.

She was still eating chocolate, but it was different. It was a conscious choice to enjoy it instead of a distraction from the issues going on inside her. That made a difference. She was capable of setting healthy boundaries and saying no to overeating or falling back into her addictive patterns. She identified her inner voices and developed compassion for herself. She also went out into nature every day. She even got to the point where she was free of physical pain. Emotionally, she was still working on a few things, but she decided she wanted a break from coaching.

She came back after a few months, and she had regained the weight. She was unhappy and frustrated, and her lower back pain came back. It was not as bad as it had been, but it was there. She was back at the beginning of her cycle. What happened? She was pulled back into the doing mode and losing herself and the deep, nourishing connection to herself. She was back in old thought patterns, trapped in her victimization, and not taking responsibility for herself. Meanwhile, she was a mom of two kids.

Her process didn't take a long time, and she was back on track more than ever. She was committed to herself and clearly taking responsibility. She developed an incredible strength and courage to speak up for herself at work, opening conflict conversations with her boss. She really claimed her authority and space. It was beautiful to witness. She was blooming from session to session. She was losing her weight again, coming back to her center, and becoming free of pain. She was back to her conscious choices of food.

These are Nadine's words:

> What I learned is that I show up at work and set my boundaries if something becomes too much. I'm voicing issues in meetings with my colleagues and bringing the issues to the table instead of withholding and internalizing anger anymore as in past times. My life has changed, and I treat and deal with my life differently. I accept what isn't changeable.
>
> I feel much freer, and I took big steps on my path to self-development and connecting with my true, authentic self and essence. I feel gratitude. Many, many thanks!
>
> I'm very proud of myself, where I stand today on my path, and how I stand in my path.

These are the moments where I feel touched and deeply moved in my heart. I love when my clients continue their inner work and stay committed to themselves, to their true paths, and feeding their new stories. I know they will keep moving toward feeling better and living pain-free lives. They will be relaxed and relieved.

Nadine asked for help when she noticed the pain coming back and returning to her old eating patterns. She wasn't waiting too long or until the pain was getting worse. Asking for help and reaching out to an expert is one way to deal with obstacles. I was very happy that Nadine scheduled a session.

I used a helpful and powerful tool to keep her focused on her new daily life. She created a vision board to keep herself focused on her new self, her new awareness, and her new life. We created a collage from pictures as a reminder and made a map. The map can be who we want to be or how we want our lives to be. It is a visual representation and a reminder of our goals, values, dreams, and visions. It is a way to teach our minds what is important to us. It can connect our subconscious wants, desires, and needs and make them conscious. A vision board can deter any big obstacles and help us connect with ourselves.

It makes me sad to see pain-free clients abandon their journeys and return to their daily lives. They think they can continue in the same way as they did before they came to me and before the pain was there. The pain is a clear sign to change your course of life and continue doing your inner work, self-mastery, and nourishment. The pain is a sign of consciousness! Every relationship starts with self-love. Continuing the inner work is necessary to feed our life stories until we transit into another life or world.

For many of my clients with lower back pain, neck pain, headaches, or other chronic pain, it was new to step into the different layers of their being, explore their being, and get in touch with their inner voices, inner children, shadows, emotions, and thought patterns. As a coach, I could view them in their process, guide them, and give them little teachings along the way. You can do it on your own by reading my book and other books or watching webinars, but it is most efficient to commit to a one-on-one program with me as your holistic and mind-set coach or participate in a group with other like-minded people and be guided and facilitated by me through your process in a group setting. You can set up the foundation and groundwork that helps you let go of pain. My coaching program opens a new dimension in your life.

There was a time in my life when I figured out everything on my own because I thought I needed to do it on my own. Unfortunately, asking for help was not on my screen at all. An old pattern kept me from moving forward. Today, I know it was more efficient to be accompanied by a coach.

As a coach, I can see, perceive, and observe your life situation from the outside better than you can when you are in a challenging situation, a painful phase, or a foggy tunnel. We are often blind to things when we are trapped or stuck in something, especially pain. Pain makes us foggy and narrows our viewpoints. I would love to help you clarify, give you new perspectives, hold you with compassion and understanding in times of exploration, and process your issues and pain.

In the meantime, here are nine steps of action:

- Ask for help and get a coach.
- Set healthy boundaries on a daily basis.
- Practice the four-steps responsibility model daily.
- Practice identifying your inner voices daily.
- Practice inner work daily.
- Practice self-mastery daily.
- Practice nourishment, self-care, and self-love daily.
- Practice rituals daily.
- Create a vision board twice a year.

Ask for help because new challenges and problems will come up after reading this book. Reach out to me via email at ab@annabelle-breuer.com. It's my pleasure to schedule a first get-to-know-each other call and listen to your situation to see if we are a good match. I promise it is much more fun and easier to work with me as your coach rather than to try to do it all on your own!

CHAPTER
12

CONCLUSION

Most people do not really want freedom, because freedom involves
responsibility, and most people are frightened of responsibility.
—Sigmund Freud

E ACH HUMAN'S JOURNEY of pain is unique, but all of my readers
and clients share the same dream: getting rid of pain and finding
relaxation, relief, and freedom from pain.

Once the decision is made—and my clients are committed to facing
their pain from another angle—the door opens to a deeper process of
consciousness, healing, transformation, and life changes. Once they decide
to take responsibility for owning their unique story of pain, the door to
freedom and pain relief opens for good.

Once they open to listening to their bodies and the messages of pain,
they get the truth about their pain and return to their essential inner truth
by changing their stories and their lives with awareness and responsibility.

The journey is the destination.
—Confucius

By choosing to trust the process and walk the talk, my clients are in
transformation. The experience and change they gain during this process
is the true reward for them.

My clients in transformation:

- want to get rid of pain and are open to experience new ways.
- are committed to themselves and want to change their stories.
- are aware of their responsibility for their lives and their bodies.
- know about physical pain, mental and emotional pain, and the relationship of the two.
- are conscious that they create their realities.
- feel their bodies and see the connection between their bodies, minds, and souls and the realities they create.
- want a safe, trustworthy container to surrender in their healing process.
- are open to letting go of old patterns, thought patterns, and beliefs that cause pain.
- are open to taking steps and changing what can be changed and accepting what can't be changed.
- are open to diving deeper into the process and exploring their inner worlds for the sake of letting go of the pain.
- are open to dreaming of their future and creating their present.

It is hard to leave you here knowing that the process has just started while reading this book. I know you are resourceful and can walk the talk on your own. However, I also know from my experience that it took much longer and was less efficient to figure it all out on my own. I avoided asking for help because of a thought pattern and a belief that I needed to work hard and figure it all out on my own. I felt shame and a bit of fear about what might happen.

Once I decided to ask for help, I met the people who supported me in my healing process and got rid of the pain. It was much more efficient, fulfilling, fun, easy, and powerful. I could not imagine how it would have been to not get the impulses from an expert and coach.

It is important for all of us to do the Shadow and Inner work and take responsibility for our own thoughts, beliefs, and emotions. We need to own them, own our stories, and return to our unique truth and soul path instead of following the lies and illusions created by our egos and unawareness. They cause separation, pain, and suffering, and we all long for connection and freedom from pain. It is necessary to consult an expert at least once in your life. A coach who is experienced in self-development will make a difference in your life, your family, your friendships, your relationships, your career, and in the world.

If you want to travel your journey on your own and do your own self-development and healing process, you can choose it. I did it partly, but it was not fun. I enjoyed traveling with somebody and having a coach who witnessed me, acknowledged me, celebrated me, held me trustworthy, held me accountable and held me with compassion and understanding. I felt safe in my process and on my roller coasters, my emotions, my feelings, and my thoughts. And it was much more fun!

Don't believe you need to do it on your own. Don't believe there's no way out of your pain situation. Don't give up. Follow and trust the process!

I hope you continue your process of healing, and I hope I meet you on the journey of getting rid of pain. I hope you escape your pain and live with freedom, joy, and compassion.

I'd love to guide your hero journey! Email me at ab@annabelle-breuer.com.

FURTHER READING

The Four Agreements by Don Miguel Ruiz
Anatomy of Peace by the Arbinger Institute
The Shaman's Body by Arnold Mindell
The Highly Sensitive Person by Elaine N. Aron, PhD
Wheels of Life by Anodea Judith, PhD
Healing Your Aloneness by Erika J. Chopich and Margaret Paul
Anatomy of the Spirit by Caroline Myss, PhD
Soul Retrieval by Sandra Ingerman
Prime-Time Health by William Sears, MD
Women's Bodies, Women's Wisdom by Christiane Northrup, MD
Dodging Energy Vampires by Christiane Northrup, MD
Red Moon by Miranda Gray

ACKNOWLEDGMENTS

SINCE EARLY CHILDHOOD, I have been very connected to nature and my body. I loved being in and with nature, and I always needed to move my body, feel my body, and be out in nature. Nature, heartfelt friends, and a connection to my body have always been a big resource for me. I'm thankful for a deep connection and belief in nature.

Growing up in a family system with dysfunctional dynamics, the experience of Shock/Developmental Trauma and being an Empath with Highly Emotional Sensitivity prepared me for life and helped me develop my psychological, spiritual, and emotional skills in addition to my holistic medical approach and worldview. This is the time to acknowledge my parents who have given me this gift of life. All the learnings with you prepared me in a way and formed me who I am and where I am today. You have always done your best as much as possible. Thank you deeply from my heart!

And a toast to my sister and my brother. I'm grateful for having you in my life! Love you both! And all my love and gratitude to my nieces, nephews and closest friends.

I was always interested in human beings. I once said, "I want to study human beings all over—from inside out and outside in." I wanted to study them holistically in all layers: physical, emotional, and mental. I'm still following this dream and studying human beings holistically because you can never stop learning. I'm grateful that I followed my intuition.

I want to thank a few people who have enriched and impacted my life with their programs and human nature. Andrew Taylor Still is the founder of osteopathy and osteopathic medicine. Arnold Mindell is the founder of process-oriented psychology. I also want to thank his wife, Amy Mindell, Kathrin Purman, my Triyoga instructor and close friend, Ashley Turner, the founder of Yoga Psychology, and Anne Weiss, Traumatherapist and expert in Shamanic Healing Rituals.

In a session with my coach, I dreamed about writing a book. Thank you, Ursula Glunk, for creating the space for me to start exploring my dream. It came up twice, and each time, it was about different content. Finally, I came across the Author Incubator, and I could fulfill my dream with Dr. Angela Laurie and her program. Thank you for creating such an amazing program. It was exactly what I needed to get the book out of me. It had been cooking inside me for a long time. My dream came true and manifested into reality.

Another shout-out and huge thank you goes to Jeanine Mancusi and Leza Danly, the founder of Lucid Living and the Great Story Coaching Program. Your program has enriched and changed my life enormously, and it has lifted my consciousness to the next level. I have always dreamed of doing quality work like that and living a life like that. Maggie Pierce, as my great story mentor coach, has supported me in exploring my great story, my love authority, and the courageous leadership connected to my soul. A big thank you goes out to you!

I want to take a moment to thank my clients and their stories I have shared in my book. I feel honored to have witnessed such hugely transformational stories and that they have chosen me as their guide on their hero's journey. I often feel like there are no words for what has happened in my clients' transformational processes. It's simply amazing. Blessings to you!

Lastly, a big thank you from deep in my heart to my husband, Okokon Udo. You're the best! Thank you for your emotional and physical support during the process of writing my first book. Thank you for encouraging me and supporting me in making this dream come true. Thank you for cheering me on and holding me powerfully, tenderly, compassionately, and critically! Thank you for believing in me and walking the path of our truest Selves together. Being married to you is fun, adventurous, and exciting. I'm grateful for our deep connection, our intimate love space, and what we have. I love you to the moon and back!

About the Author

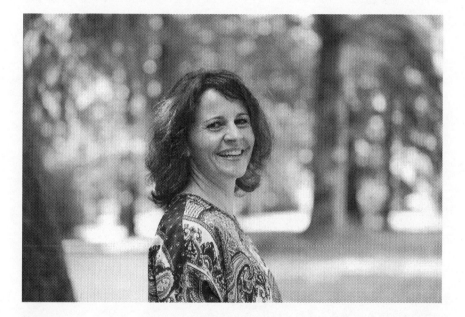

A NNABELLE BREUER-UDO MADE a career as a practitioner of osteopathic medicine, naturopath, psychotherapist, Triyoga instructor, university faculty member, workshop facilitator, and certified professional life and holistic health coach (ACC, CPCC). She is an expert in Process-Oriented Psychology and Yoga Psychology.

Before moving from Germany to the United States, she worked with physicians and hospital environments for more than two decades and was the founder and director of her practice. Annabelle's career path has been expanded through experiences and training at Co-Active Leadership,

Great Story Coaching, Process Work, Yoga Psychology, and Meditation Training at McLean Meditation Institute.

She is passionate about helping individuals with chronic stress and pain who are looking for a holistic solution that does more than just mask the pain and stress. She helps busy professionals and moms heal from chronic pain and stress, prioritize their health, and enjoy life again. She intimately understands the different levels of pain and stress and how they affect various personalities—both inside and out.

Her life coaching, holistic health coaching, compassionate guidance and holistic health approach will help you understand how your Lifestyle, Exercise, Attitude, and Nutrition choices integrate and set the stage for your overall health. Her coaching program will help you change your relationship with pain and stress and make the body-mind-soul connection to manage and heal your pain and stress in a holistic and empowering way. She will support you in making a difference in your life whether it is in your health, relationships, life transition, self-development or redefining your life's purpose.

She works with clients locally, nationally, and abroad in individual, group, virtual, and in-person sessions. She is passionate about nature, traveling, food, body-mind-spirit renewal, love, and connection. Annabelle lives happily with her husband, Okokon, in Minneapolis, Minnesota.

Website: www.annabelle-breuer.com
Email: ab@annabelle-breuer.com
Facebook: http://www.facebook.com/annabellebreuerudo
Ayurvedic Cleanse Program Description: http://annabelle-breuer.lpages.com/ayurvedic-cleanse-10-program

Thank you for reading *The Magic about Pain: How Facing Your Pain Can Transform Your Life*. I'd love to guide you on your hero's journey and support you in your process of getting rid of pain, feeling relaxed and relieved, and making health your priority.

Are you looking for the next steps? I've created a short video series to get you started on your journey. Email me at ab@annabelle-breuer.com with "The Magic about Pain" in the subject line, and I'll send you the link!